Mastering Pleasure: A Guide to Self-Discovery and Exploration

Monica Lynne Chase

Foreword

Welcome to *Mastering Pleasure: A Guide to Self-Discovery and Exploration*, a book designed to help you uncover the depths of your own pleasure and self-understanding. This isn't just about pleasure as a passing sensation; it's about learning to celebrate and connect with yourself on a deeply personal level. This journey is for everyone who has ever felt a curiosity about their own body or wondered if there is more to intimacy than what they have been told.

In this book, we will explore everything from solo sexuality and breaking taboos to creating a personal space that fosters comfort, privacy, and pleasure. Mastering Pleasure isn't just about technique; it's about empowering you to love yourself, to let go of shame, and to experience your own body and mind with respect, joy, and openness. Whether you're familiar with solo exploration or entirely new to the concept, you'll find the tools in this book to approach yourself with a fresh perspective and a sense of curiosity.

As you turn these pages, know that you are embarking on a journey that's uniquely yours. With compassion, knowledge, and a sense of discovery, this book encourages you to step beyond societal expectations and explore your pleasure and individuality. Embrace this experience with openness, celebrate each step, and, most importantly, enjoy every moment of the beautiful journey of mastering your own pleasure.

Introduction

Welcome to *Mastering Pleasure: A Guide to Self-Discovery and Exploration*—a book that invites you to understand, embrace, and celebrate your unique experience of pleasure and self-love. Many of us grow up with mixed messages about sexuality and pleasure, often conditioned by societal expectations, stigmas, and myths that can leave us feeling conflicted about our own desires and needs. This book aims to break through those barriers, offering a space where you can explore and redefine what pleasure, intimacy, and self-love mean to you.

At its core, Mastering Pleasure is about empowerment. It's about reconnecting with your body, understanding the beauty of solo sexuality, and appreciating how this self-connection contributes to your overall mental and emotional health. For many, solo pleasure is an area of life that carries shame or secrecy. Here, however, we view it as a natural, enriching practice—one that helps foster confidence, self-acceptance, and a deeper understanding of one's own needs and boundaries. Solo exploration is more than a physical act; it's a journey inward, cultivating a sense of respect for yourself and for what brings you personal joy.

This book is structured to guide you step-by-step, from creating a welcoming, comfortable space for yourself to trying out techniques that allow you to understand your body and your preferences. You'll learn about mindfulness practices that can enhance your experience and connect your mind and body, turning self-discovery into a form of meditation. We'll also address and challenge common myths, look into the powerful role of fantasy, and explore the benefits of integrating pleasure into daily life as a form of self-care and emotional balance.

In these chapters, you'll find practical tips, encouraging guidance, and a wealth of information that reframes solo pleasure as a valuable tool for growth and well-being. By the end of this journey, you'll not only feel more in tune with your body but also more equipped to navigate your emotional landscape, set healthy boundaries, and celebrate your personal needs. So let this be your VIP invitation to embark on a liberating journey of self-discovery, free from judgment and filled with curiosity. Embrace this opportunity to explore, learn, and, most importantly, enjoy every part of the experience.

Table of Contents

This table of contents guides readers through a supportive journey of self-discovery, helping them embrace their bodies, deepen their self-awareness, and celebrate the empowerment that comes with knowing and valuing their own pleasure.

Chapter 1: The Art of Self-Love

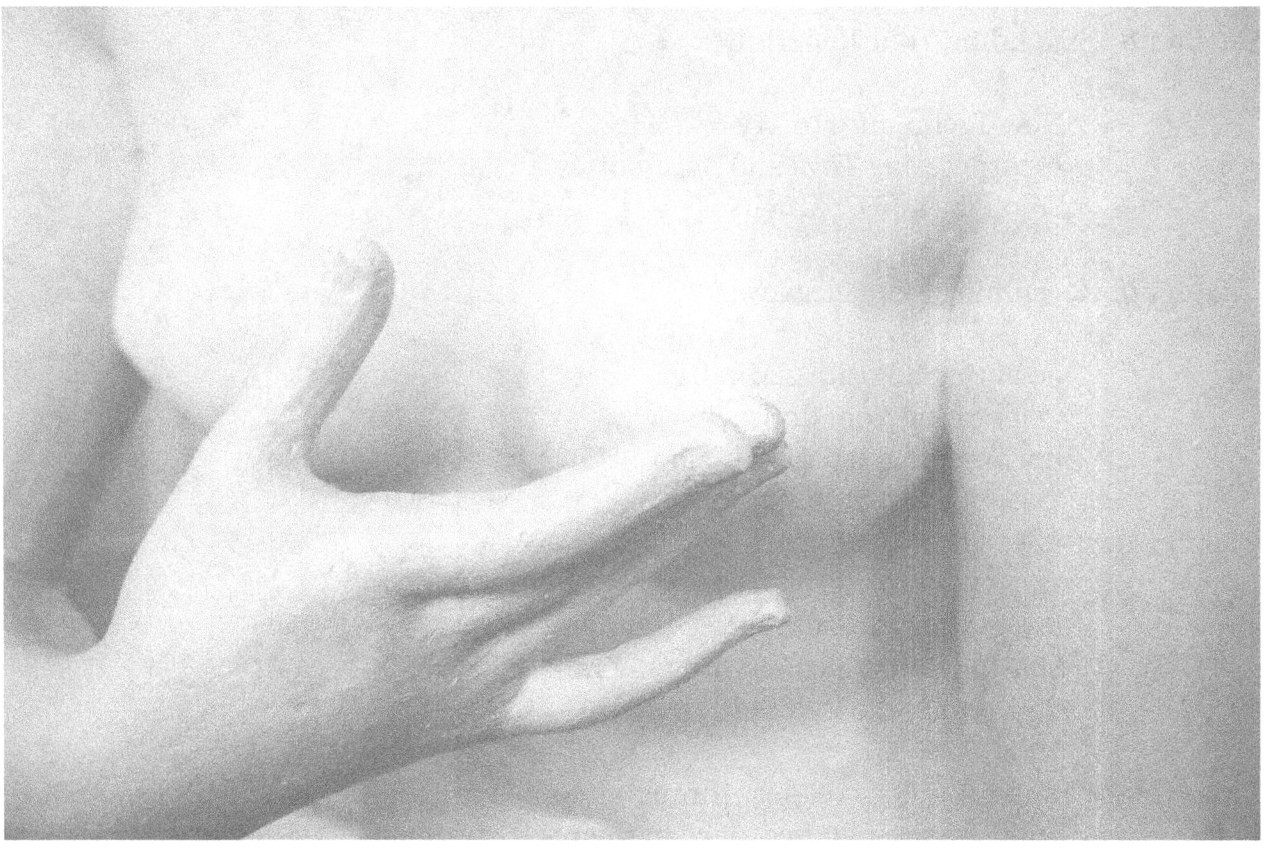

Embracing Your Body

Embracing your body is the first step on the exhilarating journey of self-discovery, and trust me, it's a journey worth taking. Our bodies are incredible vessels that hold our desires, sensations, and unique pleasures. In a world that often bombards us with unrealistic expectations and rigid ideals, it's time to break free from those constraints and celebrate our individuality. So, let's throw away the shame and embrace every curve, line, and imperfection. Your body is not just a shell; it's a playground of sensations waiting to be explored.

We often forget that self-pleasure is more than just a physical act; it's an intimate conversation between you and your body. When you take the time to engage with yourself, you're not just indulging in pleasure; you're learning what makes you tick, what ignites that spark, and what brings you joy. So, set aside any lingering doubts and allow yourself to explore every inch of your being. Touch yourself with curiosity and love, and remember that there's no right or wrong way to experience pleasure. It's all about finding what feels good for you and embracing those sensations wholeheartedly.

Breaking societal taboos around masturbation and self-pleasure is a powerful form of self empowerment. For too long, these natural and beautiful expressions of intimacy have been shrouded in guilt and secrecy. By embracing your body and your desires, you're taking a stand against those outdated notions. You're reclaiming your pleasure and asserting your right to enjoy every part of your body without shame or judgment. This reclamation is not just an act of self-love; it's a revolutionary statement that your pleasure matters and that it's time to celebrate it unapologetically.

As you delve into the world of solo sexual practices, remember that it's not just about the destination; it's about the journey. Experimentation is key! Try different techniques, explore various fantasies, and allow your imagination to run wild. From sensual massages to playful toys, indulge in whatever makes your heart race and your body tingle. The more you explore, the more you'll discover about yourself, your desires, and what truly brings you joy. It's a delightful process of trial and error, so don't be afraid to get a little messy along the way.

Embracing your body is about cultivating a loving relationship with yourself. This journey of self-discovery allows you to connect not only with your physical self but also with your mental and emotional well-being. When you prioritize your pleasure and body, you're investing in your overall happiness. This newfound confidence will radiate into other areas of your life, enhancing your intimacy with partners and enriching your sexual experiences. So, dive in, celebrate your body, and remember that every moment spent embracing yourself is a step toward mastering the art of pleasure.

The Power of Pleasure

Pleasure is a powerful force that can transform our lives in ways we often overlook. When it comes to self-pleasure, or masturbation, many people shy away from discussing it openly, but this is precisely where the magic lies. Embracing the joy of solo sexual practices allows us to reconnect with our bodies and understand what truly turns us on. It's like embarking on a treasure hunt, where the prize is self-knowledge and empowerment. So, let's dive into the delightful world of pleasure and see how it can lead us to greater intimacy with ourselves and others.

Imagine your body as a wonderland, filled with hidden paths and secret spots waiting to be explored. Self-pleasure is your ticket to this enchanting journey, where every touch can reveal something new about your desires. With each exploration, you become more attuned to your preferences, unlocking a treasure trove of sensations that can enhance your sexual experiences. It's a playful dance, an opportunity to discover your rhythm without the pressure of performance or judgment. The more you indulge in this exploration, the more you reclaim your body as a source of joy and fulfillment.

In a society that often shrouds sexuality in shame and taboo, embracing the power of pleasure becomes an act of rebellion. By celebrating self-pleasure, we challenge outdated beliefs and rewrite the narrative around intimacy. This is about empowerment—taking back control over our bodies and desires. When we break free from societal constraints, we not only enhance our own sexual lives but also pave the way for others to do the same. Together, we can create a culture that honors pleasure and encourages open conversations about what it means to truly feel good.

Now, let's talk about technique! Self-pleasure isn't just a mindless act; it's an art form waiting to be mastered. From varying your pace and pressure to experimenting with different fantasies, your solo sessions can be as dynamic as you desire. Try incorporating props, such as toys or even just a cozy blanket, to elevate your experience. Don't be afraid to get creative! The goal is to explore what feels best for you, allowing your imagination to run wild. Remember, there's no right or wrong way to enjoy yourself— only the path that leads to your unique pleasure.

Let's not forget the mental health benefits that come with embracing pleasure. Engaging in solo sexual practices can reduce stress, boost mood, and enhance overall well-being. It's like a mini-vacation for your mind and body, allowing you to unwind and reconnect. By prioritizing pleasure, we cultivate a sense of self-love and acceptance, which spills over into other areas of our lives. So, the next time you find yourself feeling guilty about indulging in self-pleasure, remind yourself that you're not just having fun; you're investing in your mental and emotional health. Celebrate your pleasure, and watch how it transforms your world!

Breaking Down Barriers

Breaking down barriers is the first step toward embracing the full spectrum of your own pleasure. In a world where societal norms often dictate what is acceptable, it's time to shake off those outdated beliefs and reclaim your right to explore your body. Masturbation isn't just a naughty secret; it's a powerful act of self-love and self-discovery. By breaking the silence around solo sexual practices, we can empower ourselves to enjoy our bodies without guilt or shame. Imagine a world where pleasure is celebrated, not hidden—let's make that world a reality together!

One of the most significant barriers to enjoying solo sexual practices is the stigma associated with masturbation. Many of us grew up with messages that painted self-exploration as something taboo, something to be whispered about or even avoided. But here's a little secret: everyone has a body, and everyone deserves to enjoy it! When you embrace masturbation as a joyful part of your life, you not only enhance your relationship with yourself but also foster a sense of empowerment. So, let's shatter those chains of societal expectations and dance freely in the realm of self-pleasure!

As we dive deeper into the art of self-exploration, it's vital to remember that pleasure comes in many forms. Whether it's through sensual touch, the thrill of experimentation, or simply enjoying the moment, the key is to listen to your body. Breaking down barriers means allowing yourself to let go of preconceived notions and embracing what truly feels good. Try new techniques, explore different sensations, and don't be afraid to get a little playful. This journey is about discovering what makes your body sing, and the only rule is to have fun along the way!

Mental health and pleasure are intricately linked, and breaking down barriers can lead to a healthier, happier you. Engaging in solo sexual practices can reduce stress, elevate your mood, and boost your confidence. It's a form of self-care that nourishes not just your body but your mind as well. When you allow yourself to indulge in pleasure, you send a powerful message to your brain: you are worthy of joy and satisfaction. So, let's embrace this connection and make self-pleasure an essential part of our mental health toolkit!

The journey to breaking down barriers is a personal one, filled with discoveries that can transform your relationship with yourself and others. By reframing how we view masturbation and solo sexual practices, we pave the way for a more open and accepting conversation about pleasure. Remember, every time you choose to indulge in self-exploration, you're contributing to the collective movement of empowerment and joy. So go ahead, break those barriers, reclaim your body, and let pleasure lead the way!

"The most intimate relationship you will ever have is the one with yourself. Cherish it, nurture it, and learn to love yourself deeply." – Anonymous

Chapter 2: Understanding Solo Sexuality

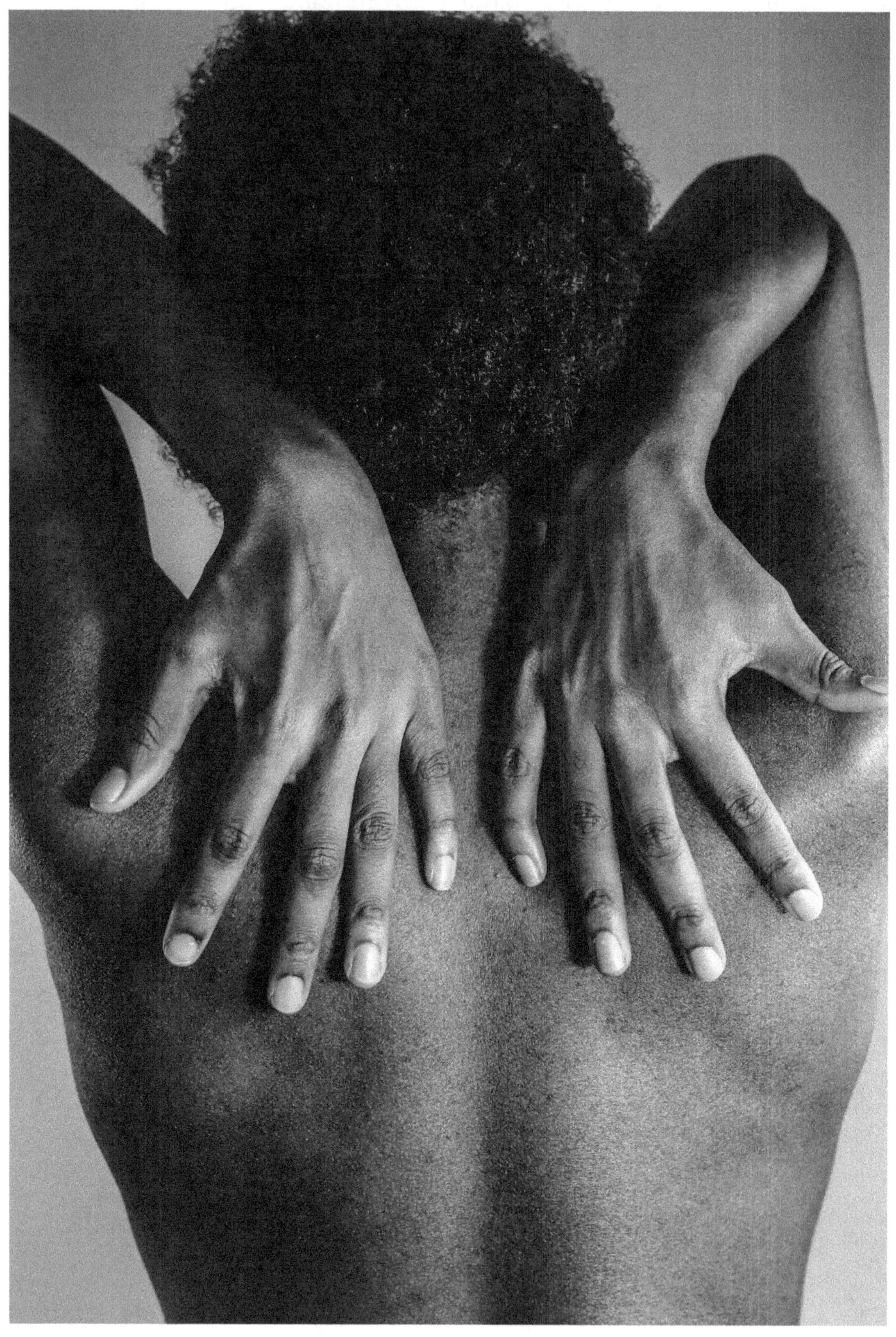

What is Solo Sexuality?

Solo sexuality is a vibrant and often overlooked aspect of human experience that invites us to explore our bodies and desires on our own terms. It encompasses the delightful journey of self-pleasure, where the focus shifts from the external to the internal, allowing individuals to connect with their own bodies in a way that is both intimate and liberating. Instead of viewing solo acts as mere substitutes for partnered sex, we can embrace them as powerful forms of self-expression and self-care. After all, who knows our bodies better than we do?

Engaging in solo sexual practices can be an incredible way to reclaim your body and pleasure. It's an opportunity to toss aside societal taboos that often paint self-pleasure in a negative light. By cultivating an attitude of playfulness and curiosity, we can turn what was once shrouded in shame into an empowering ritual. Each stroke, caress, or fantasy can be a celebration of who we are, allowing us to explore our unique desires without any pressure or judgment. This journey of self-exploration can be both enlightening and exhilarating, creating a deeper understanding of our sexual selves.

Moreover, solo sexuality can serve as a vital component of mental health. In a world that constantly bombards us with external expectations, taking time to focus on our own pleasure can be a form of self-care that promotes emotional well-being. This practice allows us to unwind, release pent-up tension, and reconnect with our bodies, fostering a sense of acceptance and love towards ourselves. When we indulge in solo sexual practices, we create a safe space where we can embrace our fantasies and desires without the need for validation from others, ultimately leading to greater self-confidence.

The art of solo sexuality also opens the door to discovering a wealth of techniques that can enhance our experiences. Whether it's exploring different forms of stimulation or incorporating toys into our routine, the possibilities are endless. This exploration can lead to profound discoveries about our bodies and what ignites our pleasure. By experimenting in a playful manner, we become the architects of our own satisfaction, gaining insights that can even enhance future intimate encounters with partners. It's all about finding what feels good for us and celebrating those moments of joy.

Solo sexuality is about embracing our individuality and taking charge of our sexual lives. It encourages us to break free from societal norms and expectations, allowing for a more authentic and fulfilling relationship with ourselves. As we delve into the world of self-pleasure, we not only enrich our own lives but also challenge the stigmas surrounding sexuality. So let's dive deep into the wondrous waters of solo sexuality, where every exploration is a step toward mastering our pleasure and nurturing our intimate selves.

The Benefits of Solo Exploration

Solo exploration is a delightful journey into your own body and desires, offering a treasure trove of benefits that go far beyond mere physical pleasure. When you embark on this solo adventure, you take the reins of your own pleasure, allowing yourself to discover what truly makes you tick. It's like being a kid in a candy store, where every nook and cranny holds the promise of sweet delights waiting to be uncovered. By embracing solo exploration, you not only learn about your body but also cultivate a deeper connection with your own sensuality.

One of the most significant benefits of solo exploration is the boost it provides to your mental health. Engaging in self-pleasure is a form of self-care that promotes relaxation and reduces stress. In a world that often feels overwhelming, taking time to explore your body can be a grounding experience. The endorphins released during these moments of bliss can elevate your mood and create a sense of euphoria, making it an essential tool for managing anxiety and enhancing your overall well-being. Think of it as a mini-vacation from the chaos of everyday life, where the only itinerary is your own pleasure.

Reclaiming your body through solo exploration is also a powerful act of empowerment. Society often imposes unrealistic standards and taboos around sexuality, leading many to feel disconnected from their own desires. By choosing to explore yourself solo, you break free from these constraints and redefine what pleasure means to you. This act of self-discovery fosters a sense of agency over your own body, transforming the way you view intimacy and connection. You become the author of your own pleasure narrative, crafting experiences that are uniquely yours, filled with joy and authenticity.

Moreover, solo exploration serves as a stepping stone to enhancing intimacy in all aspects of your life. The more you understand your own desires, the better equipped you are to communicate them with partners. It's like learning the ropes of a new dance; once you know the moves, you can invite someone else to join you on the floor. This understanding fosters deeper connections, as you become more confident in expressing your needs and preferences. The result? A more fulfilling sexual experience, whether you're solo or sharing that intimacy with someone special.

Let's not overlook the incredible variety of techniques and sensations that solo exploration can introduce into your sexual life. From experimenting with different rhythms to discovering new erogenous zones, each session can be a fresh adventure that keeps your pleasure repertoire exciting. Think of it as a treasure map to your own sensuality, where each exploration leads to new discoveries and delights. So, grab your favorite tools, set the mood, and dive into a world where your pleasure reigns supreme. Embracing solo exploration is not just about self-pleasure; it's about celebrating the unique, beautiful, and empowering journey of discovering yourself.

The Myths and Misconceptions

When it comes to solo sexual practices and masturbation, the landscape is littered with myths and misconceptions that can make even the most adventurous spirits hesitate. One common myth is that masturbation is somehow "bad" or "dirty." This notion often stems from outdated beliefs and societal taboos that have been passed down through generations. In reality, masturbation is a natural and healthy expression of sexuality. It's a safe space for exploration where you can learn what brings you pleasure without the pressures or complexities of a partner. So go ahead and embrace your inner pleasure enthusiast—there's nothing wrong with a little self-love!

Another misconception is that masturbation is only for those who are single or lacking intimacy. Some people might think that indulging in self-pleasure signals a deficiency in sexual relationships, but that's simply not true! Many people in fulfilling relationships use masturbation as an opportunity to enhance their sexual experiences. It can help you understand your body better and communicate your desires more effectively to your partner. Plus, self-pleasure can be a delightful way to unwind—allowing you to explore your fantasies and desires, even when you're not in the mood for a partner's company.

Many believe that there's a "right" way to masturbate, leading to feelings of inadequacy or confusion. This myth can create unnecessary pressure and detract from the joy of exploration. The truth is, there is no one-size-fits-all technique for self-pleasure. What feels amazing for one person might not resonate with another, and that's perfectly okay! The key is to experiment with different techniques and find out what makes your body sing. Whether it's using your hands, toys, or even just your imagination, the journey of discovery is as important as the destination.

Some people worry that masturbation could lead to addiction or negatively impact their sex life. While it's true that anything can be overdone, self-pleasure is generally a healthy part of a balanced sexual life. It's all about moderation and understanding your own needs. If you notice that masturbation is interfering with your daily life or relationships, it might be worth exploring those feelings further. But for the majority, it's a wonderful way to connect with your body and release pent-up energy. So, let go of that fear and enjoy the ride!

Let's address the myth that masturbation is solely a physical act. While it certainly has physical benefits—like reducing stress and enhancing sexual function—there's also a deeply emotional and mental aspect to it. Engaging in solo sexual practices can empower you, boost your self-esteem, and promote a positive body image. It's an opportunity to reclaim your pleasure, set the stage for intimacy, and ultimately embrace the beautiful complexity of your own sexuality. So, break free from the chains of outdated beliefs and misconceptions, and revel in the delightful world of self-discovery that awaits you!

"To know yourself, to honor your body and mind, is to unlock a lifetime of empowerment and self-love." – Monica Lynne Chase

Chapter 3: Creating Your Pleasure Space

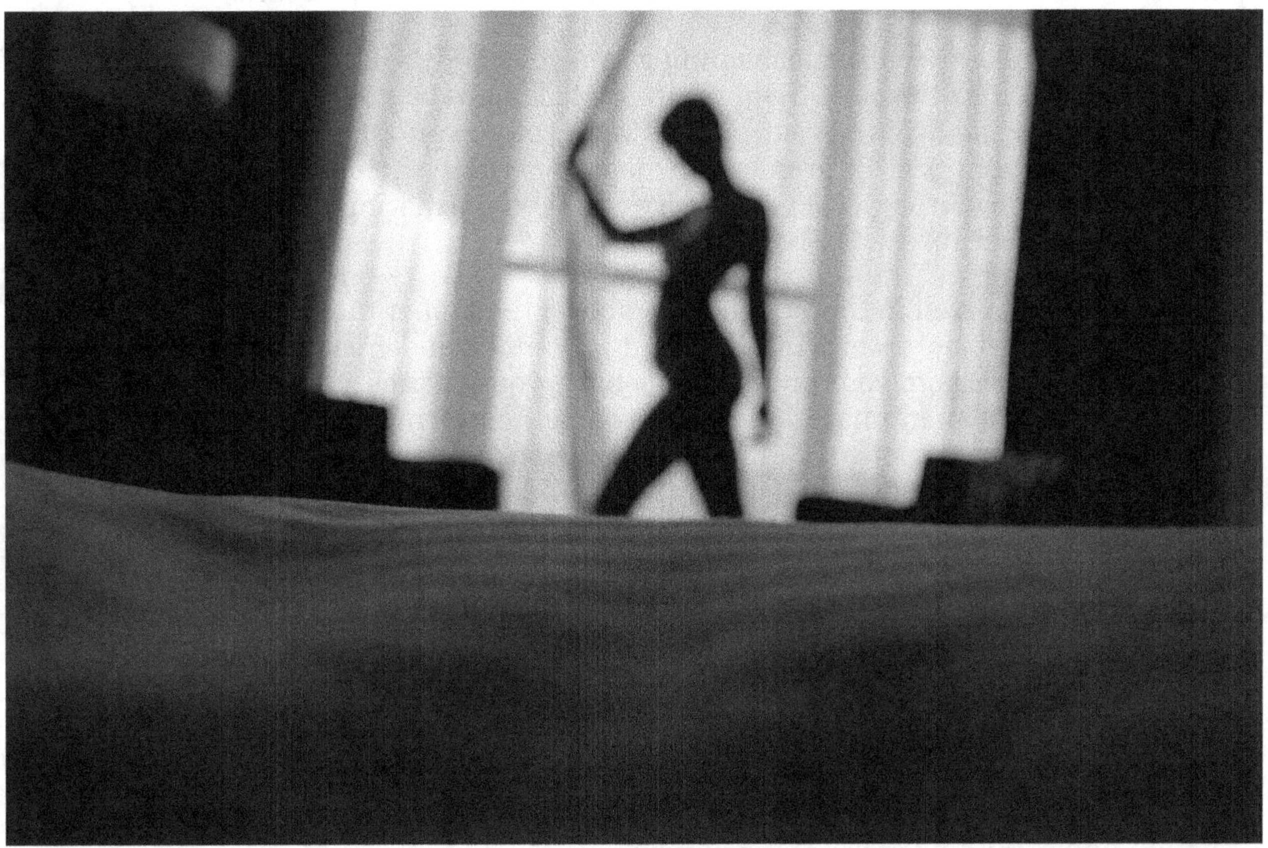

Setting the Mood

Creating the perfect ambiance for self-exploration is essential in setting the mood for your solo adventures. Think of your space as a sanctuary where you can freely express your desires without judgment. Dim the lights or light some candles to create a warm glow that invites relaxation. Soft music in the background can act as a delightful soundtrack to your journey, enhancing the sensations you're about to experience. Remember, this is your time to connect with yourself, so let go of distractions and focus on crafting an environment that feels safe and inviting.

Next, consider the power of scent. Aromatherapy can significantly elevate your mood and stimulate your senses. Choose essential oils or candles with fragrances that resonate with you—perhaps lavender for relaxation, or something fruity to spark excitement. As you breathe in these delightful scents, allow them to envelop you, making every inhale a step deeper into your pleasure zone. Your senses are your allies in this journey of self-discovery, so indulge them fully.

Now, let's talk about the playful side of self-exploration. This is your chance to embrace your inner child and experiment without pressure or expectations. Bring out toys, props, or even playful accessories that ignite your imagination. Whether it's a feather, a soft blindfold, or a favorite piece of clothing, these elements can enhance your experience, turning it into an adventure of exploration. Allow yourself to be curious and spontaneous; after all, there are no rules when it comes to your pleasure.

Engaging in self-pleasure also means tuning into your body's needs and desires. Take a moment to check in with yourself—how are you feeling today? What kind of touch feels good? Slow down and listen to your body as you explore various techniques. You might find that varying your pace or pressure opens new pathways to pleasure. Be playful in your approach; the journey of self-discovery is all about experimentation and finding what makes you feel alive.

As you immerse yourself in this delightful practice, remember that embracing your sexuality is an act of empowerment. By setting the mood and creating a sacred space for self-pleasure, you reclaim your body and celebrate your desires. This is not just about physical release; it's an intimate dance with yourself, fostering a deeper connection to your mind and body. So, let go of inhibitions, revel in the joy of self-exploration, and embrace the beautiful journey of mastering your pleasure.

Choosing the Right Tools

When it comes to the delightful journey of self-exploration, selecting the right tools can elevate your experience from ordinary to extraordinary. In the realm of solo sexual practices, these tools can range from simple household items to specialized devices designed to enhance pleasure. The key is to embrace curiosity and allow yourself to explore what resonates with your body and desires. Think of this as your personal treasure hunt, where the ultimate prize is a deeper connection with yourself and a more profound understanding of your own pleasure.

First on the list are the classics: your hands. These versatile tools are always at your disposal and can be your best friends in the quest for pleasure. Experiment with different strokes, pressures, and rhythms. Use your fingertips to tease and explore sensitive areas, or let your palms glide smoothly over your skin. The beauty of using your hands is that they can adapt to your mood and desires, making them the perfect starting point for your solo sessions. Remember, there are no rules here—only what feels good to you.

If you're ready to take things up a notch, consider incorporating sex toys into your routine. The market is bursting with a variety of options, from vibrators to dildos, each designed to cater to different preferences and fantasies. Don't be afraid to explore! Vibrators can introduce exciting sensations that you may not achieve with just your hands. Try out various shapes, sizes, and functions to find what tickles your fancy. The right toy can become a trusty companion in your adventures, helping you break free from the confines of societal taboos and empowering you to reclaim your pleasure.

For those who enjoy a little extra creativity, household items can also serve as surprising tools for your exploration. Think of items that are safe, clean, and have interesting textures or shapes. A soft cloth, a warm towel, or even a showerhead can add new dimensions to your pleasure journey. Just remember to prioritize safety and ensure that whatever you choose is body-safe and clean. The goal is to unleash your imagination while keeping your exploration enjoyable and risk-free.

Don't underestimate the power of ambiance in your self-pleasure sessions. Creating a comfortable and inviting space can enhance your experience significantly. Consider lighting some candles, playing your favorite music, or using essential oils for a sensory delight. The right environment can help you relax and fully immerse yourself in the moment. By choosing the right tools, both physical and environmental, you set the stage for an empowering and pleasurable exploration of your body—one that not only nourishes your mental health but also encourages you to celebrate your sexuality without shame.

Privacy and Comfort

Privacy and comfort are the cozy blankets that wrap around your self-exploration journey, creating a safe haven where you can truly connect with your body and desires. When it comes to mastering self-pleasure, these elements are non-negotiable. Think of privacy as your sacred space, where the outside world fades away, and it's just you and your inner world. Whether it's a dimly lit room, a secluded corner of your home, or a cozy bubble bath, finding that perfect spot allows your mind to relax and your senses to awaken. Give yourself permission to create a sanctuary that invites exploration without judgment or interruption.

Comfort, on the other hand, is all about ensuring that you're physically and emotionally at ease. This might mean wearing your favorite soft pajamas, lighting a scented candle, or playing some soothing music that makes your heart flutter. It's essential to tune into what feels good for you—what allows your body to release tension and embrace pleasure. Remember, the journey of self-discovery is not just about the destination but also about enjoying every moment along the way. When you prioritize comfort, you're sending a loving message to your body that it deserves to be cherished and celebrated.

Now, let's talk about the delightful dance of boundaries. Establishing privacy means setting clear boundaries, not just with others but also with yourself. It's honoring your time, your space, and your feelings. This could be as simple as turning off your phone notifications or letting housemates know you need some "me time." Think of it as putting up a cozy "Do Not Disturb" sign, inviting only the most pleasurable thoughts and sensations. When you carve out this time for self-exploration, you're empowering yourself to dive deep into the ocean of your desires without the waves of distraction crashing in.

Creating an atmosphere of privacy and comfort also helps dismantle societal taboos surrounding self-pleasure. When you feel secure in your private space, you can fully embrace the joy of exploring your body and your fantasies. This is an act of rebellion against a world that often shames us for our desires. So, let's shatter those stereotypes! As you delve into your solo sexual practices, remind yourself that this exploration is not just a means of pleasure; it's a celebration of empowerment and reclaiming your body. Each moment spent in your sanctuary is a step toward embracing who you are and what you want.

Also, remember that privacy and comfort are your allies in the pursuit of self-pleasure. They help you tune into your body's rhythms, discover what makes you tick, and ignite your passions. As you embark on this journey of self-discovery, let these elements be your guiding stars. Embrace the freedom to explore, the joy of comfort, and the power of privacy, and you'll find yourself not only mastering pleasure but also celebrating the beautiful, intricate relationship you have with yourself. Enjoy the ride, and let the magic unfold!

"The journey to self-love and self-acceptance begins by honoring your own needs, desires, and worth." – Lalah Delia

Chapter 4: Techniques for Self-Discovery

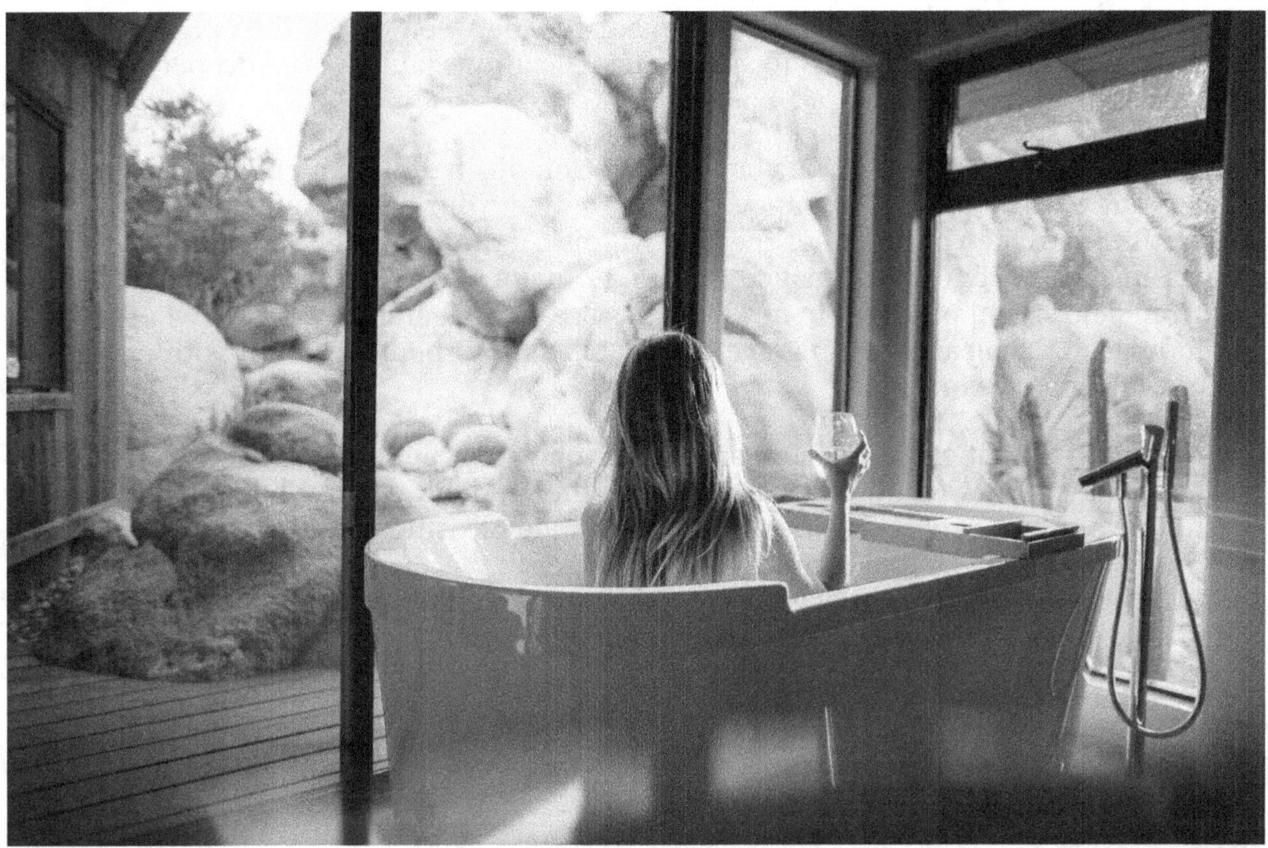

Exploring Sensation

Exploring sensation is the thrilling adventure we embark on when we decide to turn our attention inward and discover the wonders of our own bodies. Imagine a world where every touch, caress, and stroke becomes an exquisite exploration of pleasure, where your fingertips become the keys to unlocking a symphony of sensations. It's time to throw off the shackles of societal expectations and delve into the treasure trove of delight that is your own body. Embrace this journey with a playful spirit, as the path to self-discovery is paved with curiosity and joy.

Start by creating a sensory-rich environment that invites exploration. Dim the lights, light some candles, or play soft music that resonates with your soul. Allow your imagination to run wild as you set the stage for a delightful rendezvous with yourself. Experiment with different textures, temperatures, and scents. Wrap yourself in silk or indulge in the warmth of a cozy blanket. Let the world around you fade as you focus on the exquisite sensations that arise from every deliberate movement. Remember, this is your time to play, and there are no rules other than the ones you create.

As you dive deeper into sensation, consider the power of touch. Your hands are not just tools; they are instruments of pleasure waiting to be played. Explore different techniques—gentle strokes, firm pressure, or tantalizing teasing. Take your time and pay attention to how your body responds. Discover the areas that make you shiver with delight and those that spark your curiosity. Each exploration is an invitation to learn more about what you enjoy, breaking down barriers between your mind and body. This playful experimentation can lead to surprising revelations and an even deeper connection with yourself.

Don't shy away from the power of your imagination during this exploration. Fantasies can be your greatest allies in enhancing sensation. Let your mind wander to the scenarios that excite you, whether they are whimsical or downright naughty. By harnessing the power of your imagination, you can amplify your physical sensations and take your solo sexual practices to new heights. Create a mental playground where you can indulge in the pleasures you crave, and watch as your body responds with electrifying enthusiasm.

This journey is about empowerment and reclaiming your pleasure. Society may have tried to dictate how we should feel about our bodies and our desires, but you are the master of your own experience. Celebrate the unique pleasures that make you who you are, and let go of any guilt or shame that may linger in the shadows. Embrace the joy of sensation as an essential part of your mental health and intimacy, not just with yourself but in all your relationships. By exploring sensation with a playful heart, you open the door to a world of pleasure that is yours and yours alone.

Rhythm and Movement

Rhythm and movement are the heartbeat of self-pleasure, transforming what could be a simple act into a vibrant dance of discovery. When you think about rhythm, consider not just the physical aspect, but also the emotional and mental pulse that runs through your experience. Whether you're swaying your hips, rolling your shoulders, or finding that perfect groove, the way your body moves can elevate your pleasure to new heights. Let your body lead, and soon you'll find that each motion can unlock a different layer of joy, inviting you to explore the delightful landscape of your own desires.

Think about the music that sets the tone for your solo adventures. Just as a great playlist can ignite your spirit, the rhythm of your movements can be equally transformative. Explore the beats that resonate with you, whether it's a sultry jazz tune or an upbeat dance track. As the music fills the space around you, let it inspire your body to sway and pulse in time. Feel the connection between sound and sensation, allowing the rhythm to guide your hands and hips, creating a symphony of pleasure that only you can compose.

Movement isn't just about the physical; it's also about being present in your body. When you engage in self-pleasure, take a moment to check in with yourself. Notice how your body feels, the sensations that arise with each caress, and the energy that flows through you. This mindfulness enhances your experience, allowing you to explore what feels right, what brings you joy, and what excites you. By tuning in to your body's natural rhythm, you can discover new techniques and practices that resonate with your desires, turning self-exploration into an empowering ritual of self-love.

Let's not forget the playful aspect of movement! Self-pleasure is an opportunity to embrace your inner child and explore your body with a sense of curiosity and joy. Don't be afraid to experiment with different positions, strokes, and speeds. Try rolling around on your bed, or maybe even dancing a little before diving into your intimate exploration. The key is to have fun and let go of any inhibitions. Remember, this is your space—there are no wrong moves when it comes to finding your groove!

Ultimately, rhythm and movement in self-pleasure are about celebrating your autonomy and reclaiming your body. In a world that often imposes rigid norms around sexuality, embracing your unique rhythm can be a radical act of self-empowerment. Allow yourself the freedom to explore, to discover what makes you feel alive, and to revel in the joy of your own pleasure. As you dance to the beat of your own drum, you're not just mastering your pleasure; you're also cultivating a deeper connection with yourself, paving the way for a richer, more fulfilling sexual life.

The Role of Fantasy

In the delightful realm of self-exploration, fantasy serves as a vibrant playground for the mind. It's the stage where your imagination can run wild, free from the constraints of reality. Fantasy allows you to explore desires that might feel taboo or simply too daring to express in everyday life. Whether it's envisioning a romantic getaway with a mythical lover or indulging in a scenario that sparks your deepest cravings, these mental escapades can enhance your solo sexual practices. Embracing your fantasies isn't just fun; it's a powerful way to connect with your desires and understand what truly makes you tick.

Engaging in fantasy while exploring your body can amplify your pleasure in surprising ways. When you let your imagination take the lead, you create a world where you can experiment with different scenarios and roles. This can introduce exciting variations into your masturbation routine. Picture yourself as the star of your own steamy movie, complete with a thrilling plot twist that keeps you on the edge of your seat. By allowing yourself to daydream, you can discover new techniques and approaches to pleasure that you may never have considered before. Suddenly, your solo sessions transform into an adventurous exploration, where every twist and turn leads you closer to ecstasy.

Mental health and pleasure are intertwined in a beautiful dance, and fantasy plays a crucial role in this relationship. When you indulge in your fantasies, you're not just seeking pleasure; you're also nurturing your mental well-being. Imagining fulfilling scenarios can serve as an escape from stress and anxiety, providing a safe space for self-expression. It's a reminder that your mind holds the keys to unlocking pleasure, even during tough times. By weaving fantasy into your intimate moments, you cultivate a positive mindset that celebrates your body and its capabilities, allowing you to reclaim your pleasure without hesitation.

Breaking societal taboos surrounding sex and pleasure is essential for personal empowerment. Fantasy offers a unique avenue for this rebellion. By embracing and exploring fantasies that society might deem inappropriate, you challenge the narratives that limit your sexual expression. This act of defiance can be liberating, allowing you to redefine your relationship with pleasure on your own terms. Every time you indulge in a fantasy, you're making a statement: your desires are valid, and they deserve to be explored. This process not only enriches your sexual life but also contributes to a broader cultural shift toward acceptance and understanding of diverse sexual expressions.

The role of fantasy in your journey of self-discovery and pleasure is one of joy and enlightenment. It invites you to be playful, to dream, and to explore without judgment. As you navigate the intricacies of solo sexual practices, let your fantasies be a guiding light, illuminating paths you may have overlooked. Whether it's a whimsical daydream or a deeply rooted desire, every fantasy adds a new layer to your understanding of pleasure. So, dive in, let your imagination soar, and embrace the enchanting world of fantasy as you master the beautiful art of self-pleasure.

"Self-love is not a destination; it's a daily commitment to nurture, honor, and celebrate who you are." – Brendon Burchard

Chapter 5: Mindfulness and Masturbation

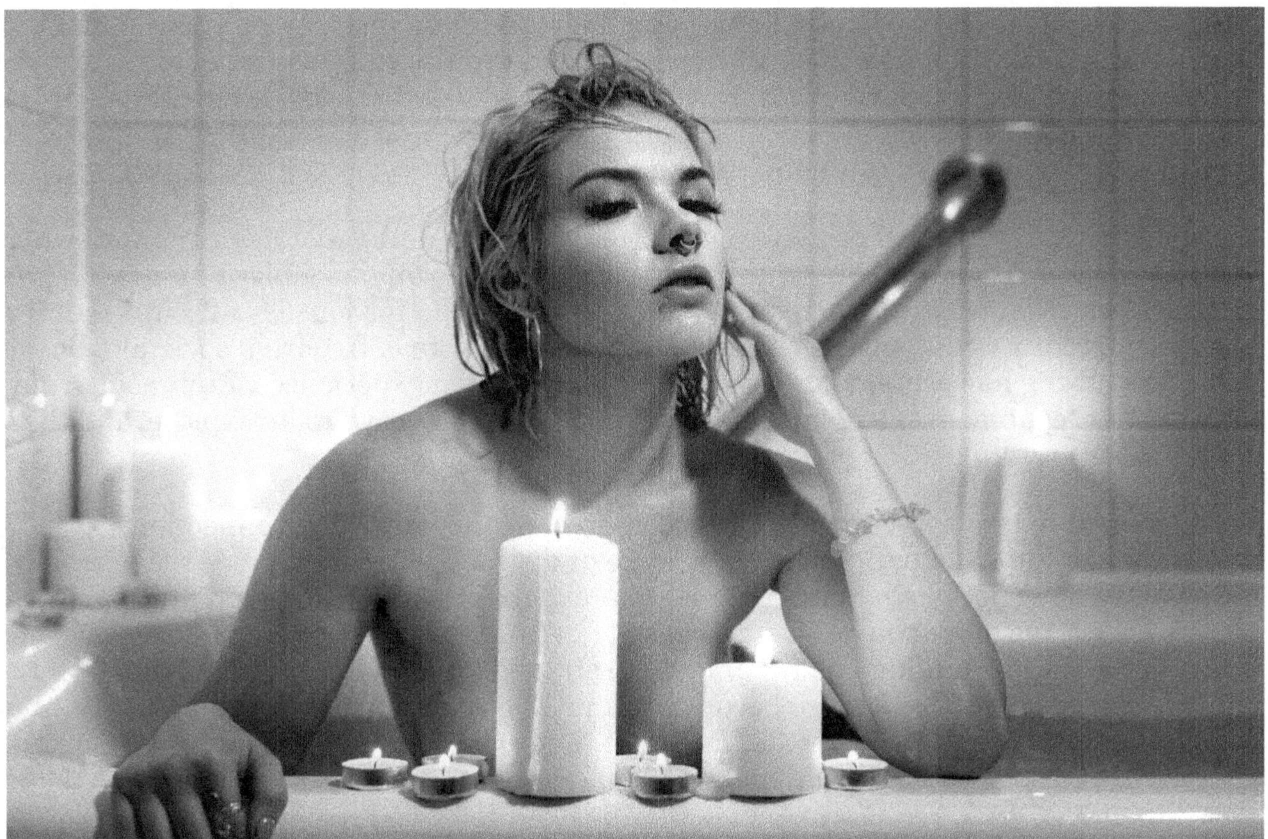

Being Present in the Moment

Being present in the moment is like discovering a hidden treasure chest within yourself, filled to the brim with delightful pleasures waiting to be explored. When it comes to self-pleasure and solo sexual practices, the first step toward unlocking the magic is to fully immerse yourself in the experience. Imagine setting the stage for your own private performance, where every sensation, every thought, and every breath becomes a part of the grand show. By tuning into the here and now, you can turn your intimate time into a rich, multi-sensory adventure that leaves you feeling empowered and deeply connected to your body.

To truly embrace presence, it's essential to shed the distractions of the outside world. This means setting the scene in a way that invites relaxation and focus. Dim the lights, light some candles, or play your favorite tunes; whatever it takes to create an atmosphere where you can shed the weight of societal expectations. By allowing yourself to be fully present, you can explore the contours of your body, the rhythm of your breath, and the sensations that arise with each touch. This is your time to experiment without judgment, to discover what makes you tick, and to indulge in the sheer joy of being you.

Mindfulness plays a pivotal role in enhancing your self-pleasure practices. By cultivating a mindful approach, you can transform what might once have felt like a hurried routine into a sacred ritual. Focus on your breathing; let it guide you deeper into your body. Notice the textures, temperatures, and sensations as they unfold. Instead of rushing towards an end goal, savor the journey. This shift in mindset not only intensifies your pleasure but also helps you to reconnect with your body, allowing you to reclaim your pleasure in a way that feels authentic and fulfilling.

Engaging in this practice of presence also fosters a deeper understanding of your desires and boundaries. As you explore your body with intention, you may uncover new fantasies or preferences that you didn't even know existed. This journey of self-discovery is a powerful form of empowerment, encouraging you to break free from societal taboos that often dictate how we should feel about our own sexual experiences. Embracing your pleasure in the moment is a bold declaration that your body is yours to explore, and that your pleasure is valid and worthy of celebration.

Being present in the moment allows you to appreciate the incredible connection between your mind and body. When you let go of distractions and embrace the here and now, you create a flow state that amplifies your experiences. The more you practice being present, the more you cultivate a sense of intimacy with yourself that spills over into other areas of your life. You become more attuned to your emotions and desires, and as a result, your self-pleasure becomes not just an act but a celebration of your whole self. So, take a deep breath, let the world fade away, and dive into the exquisite pleasure that awaits you in the moment.

Breathwork and Relaxation

Breathwork is like the secret ingredient in the recipe of self-exploration and pleasure. Imagine diving deep into a world where your breath becomes your guide, leading you to uncharted territories of relaxation and joy. By simply tuning into your breath, you can unlock the doors to heightened sensations and deeper connections with your body. It's not just a tool for relaxation; it's your personal invitation to explore the delightful realm of self-pleasure. So, let's take a moment to inhale the good vibes and exhale any tension that might be lingering, allowing ourselves to be fully present in the experience.

As you settle into your space, begin with a few deep breaths. Inhale slowly through your nose, filling your belly like a balloon, and then gently release the air through your mouth. This rhythmic flow not only calms the mind but also awakens your senses, making every touch feel electric. When you're in a relaxed state, your body becomes a playground for pleasure. Each breath can act as a soft caress, guiding you to discover what feels good. You might find that focusing on your breath transforms routine moments into sacred rituals of self-love and exploration.

Breathwork can also serve as a bridge to connecting your body and mind. When you breathe intentionally, you create a space where you can tune into your emotions and physical sensations. This connection is vital when embracing solo sexual practices or masturbation techniques. Instead of rushing through the experience, let your breath slow you down, allowing pleasure to build gradually. Picture each inhale as a wave of energy rising within you and each exhale as a release of any inhibitions or societal taboos that might be holding you back. The more you practice this, the more you'll find yourself in a state of empowerment and liberation.

Incorporating breathwork into your intimate moments can transform your entire experience. When you feel the urge to explore your body, try pausing and taking a few deep breaths first. Notice how this simple act can heighten your awareness of every sensation, every curve, and every heartbeat. You might discover new erogenous zones or techniques that bring you profound pleasure. The playful dance between breath and sensation encourages a sense of curiosity and experimentation; after all, this journey is all about reclaiming your body and your pleasure.

Breathwork isn't just about relaxation; it's about embracing the fullness of your experience. It invites you to be present, to savor each moment, and to connect deeply with your desires. As you master the art of breath and pleasure, you'll find a newfound confidence in your solo practices. So go ahead, take a deep breath, and dive into the world of self-discovery. Let your breath lead the way as you explore the delicious possibilities that await you.

Connecting Mind and Body

Imagine your mind and body as the ultimate power couple, ready to take on the world of pleasure together. When you connect these two entities, you unlock a treasure trove of sensations and experiences that can elevate your solo sexual practices to new heights. It's not just about the physical act; it's about creating a harmonious relationship between your thoughts, emotions, and body. By tapping into this connection, you can enhance your self-pleasure routines, making them not only more satisfying but also a profound journey of self-discovery.

To get started, let's embrace the idea that your body is a playground and your mind is the curator of fun. Begin with a few moments of mindfulness—perhaps a gentle stretch, some deep breathing, or even a little dance. As you engage your body in these delightful activities, pay attention to the sensations that arise. Notice how your thoughts might wander, and gently guide them back to the present moment. This practice not only grounds you but also fosters a deeper awareness of how your body responds to different stimuli. The more in tune you become with your physical sensations, the more thrilling your self-exploration can be.

Now, let's talk about the power of imagination. Your mind is a canvas, and your fantasies are the colors that paint your pleasure. As you settle into your self-pleasure practice, allow your thoughts to roam free. Create vivid scenarios that excite you, whether it's reliving a romantic moment, envisioning a playful encounter, or exploring new fantasies. This mental stimulation can heighten your arousal and transform an ordinary experience into something extraordinary. Remember, there are no limits in your imagination; this is your time to break free from societal taboos and embrace your desires without judgment.

In the world of self-exploration, using your body as a tool for pleasure can be an empowering experience. Experiment with different techniques, rhythms, and pressures, all while tuning into your body's responses. What feels good? What makes you sigh with delight? By connecting your mental desires with physical exploration, you can discover new pathways to pleasure. Don't shy away from mixing in your favorite toys or trying out different settings—perhaps dimming the lights or playing your favorite playlist. Each element contributes to the overall experience, creating a rich tapestry of sensations that can leave you breathless.

Celebrate the joy of connecting your mind and body by practicing gratitude for your unique journey. Acknowledge each time you explore, each moment you embrace your pleasure, and each step you take toward reclaiming your body. This celebration reinforces the bond between mind and body, creating a cycle of empowerment that fuels your self-discovery. Remember, mastering pleasure is not just a destination; it's an ongoing adventure filled with playful exploration, emotional connection, and the joyful reclamation of your desires. So, go ahead—dive in, play around, and savor every delightful moment!

"Pleasure is not a luxury; it is a profound gift to yourself and an essential part of your journey toward wholeness." – Alexandra Roxo

Chapter 6: Breaking Taboos and Societal Norms

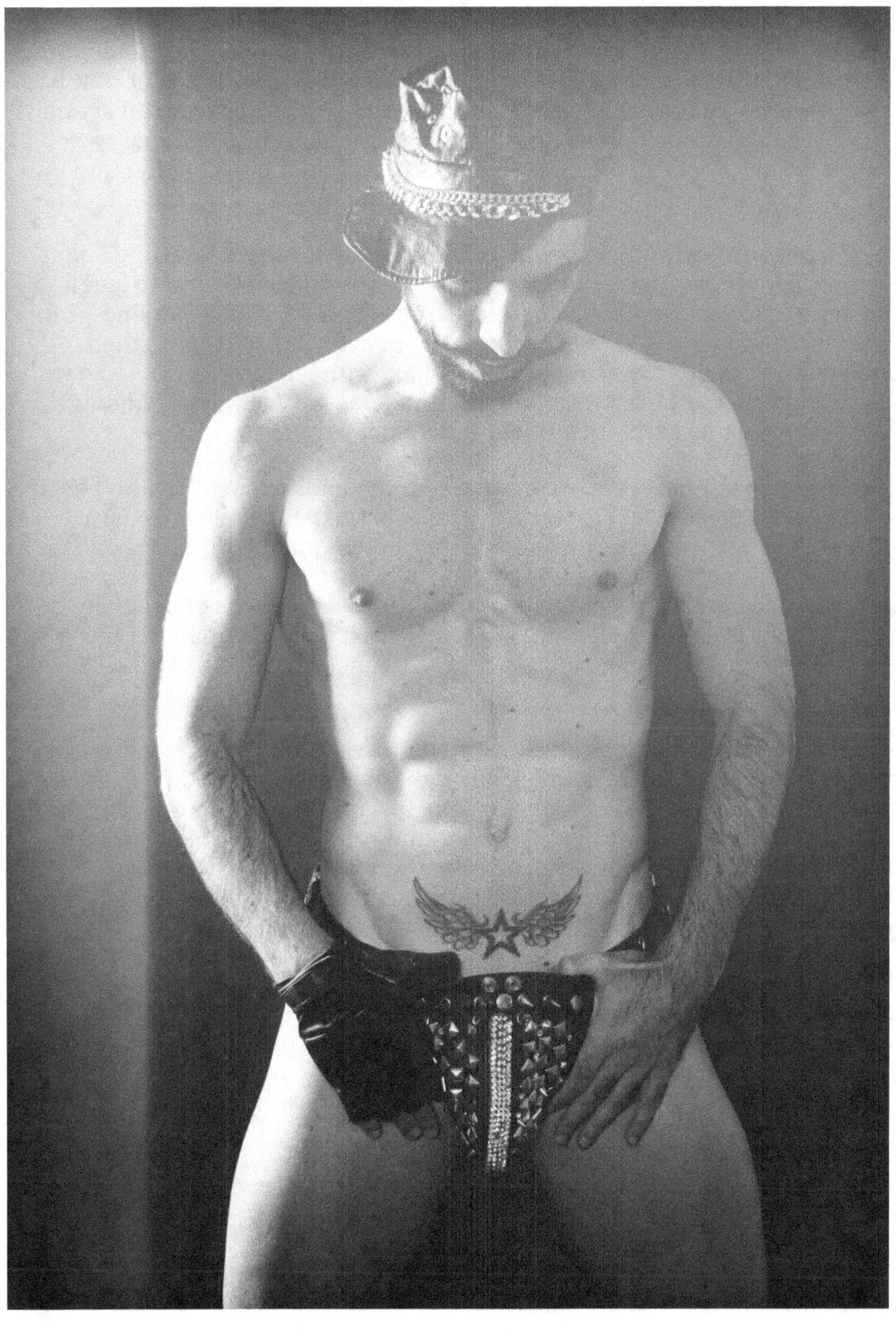

Challenging Stigmas

Challenging stigmas around self-pleasure is an exhilarating journey that invites us to shake off outdated beliefs and embrace our bodies with joy. For too long, societal norms have wrapped masturbation in a cloak of shame, relegating it to a guilty secret. But let's flip the script! Masturbation is a celebration of self-love and empowerment, an act that not only ignites physical pleasure but also fosters a deeper connection with our own desires. The more we talk about it, the less taboo it becomes, and the more liberated we feel to explore our bodies without judgment.

Imagine a world where discussing solo sexual practices is as normal as chatting about our favorite snacks. How liberating would it be to share tips on techniques, to laugh about the sometimes awkward moments, or to celebrate those blissful experiences? By openly challenging the stigma, we create a safe space for everyone to express their curiosities and preferences. It's time to replace whispers with laughter, and shame with confidence. Let's embrace our quirks, our fantasies, and our unique ways of finding pleasure, all while supporting each other in our individual journeys.

As we delve deeper into self-discovery, we inevitably confront the mental health benefits that come with mastering self-pleasure. Engaging in solo sexual practices can be a marvelous stress reliever, a way to reconnect with our bodies amidst the chaos of life. When we give ourselves permission to indulge in pleasure, we release endorphins and reduce anxiety, transforming our mental landscapes into vibrant fields of positivity. Let's make it clear: prioritizing our pleasure is not selfish; it's an essential part of maintaining our overall well-being, a radical act of self-care that deserves to be celebrated.

Breaking societal taboos surrounding self-pleasure requires courage and creativity. It's about reframing the narrative and reclaiming our right to experience joy in our own bodies. Picture this: instead of feeling shame, we can feel pride in our ability to explore our desires, to learn what brings us joy, and to communicate those needs in our intimate relationships. This reclamation is powerful, a declaration that our pleasure matters, and that we have the agency to define it on our own terms. Let's challenge the myths together and turn the conversation into one of empowerment and joy.

In this playful exploration of self-pleasure, let's also embrace the art of experimenting with techniques that suit our unique rhythms and preferences. From tantalizing teases to blissful releases, there's a vast playground waiting to be explored. Every individual is a masterpiece, and discovering what makes us tick is part of the fun. So, let's share our discoveries, learn from one another, and cultivate a culture of exploration and acceptance. In doing so, we not only enrich our sexual lives but also pave the way for a more open and accepting world where everyone can feel empowered to master their own pleasure.

Celebrating Diversity in Pleasure

Celebrating diversity in pleasure is like throwing a vibrant party where everyone is invited to explore, express, and embrace their unique desires. Pleasure isn't a one-size-fits-all experience; it's a colorful tapestry woven from the threads of our individual preferences, fantasies, and identities. Whether you're a seasoned explorer of solo sexual practices or just dipping your toes into the world of self-pleasure, understanding and celebrating what makes your pleasure unique can unlock new levels of joy and fulfillment.

Imagine your pleasure as a buffet of delightful options, each dish representing a different facet of your sensuality. Some might savor the gentle caress of a feather, while others might lean towards the exhilarating thrill of a firmer touch. By experimenting with various techniques, you can discover what tantalizes your senses and ignites your passion. Don't shy away from trying out different toys, techniques, or even fantasies that dare to push your boundaries. Each new experience is an invitation to learn more about your body and what truly brings you joy, making self-discovery a delicious adventure.

Breaking societal taboos surrounding masturbation and self-pleasure is vital in creating a culture where diversity in pleasure is not only accepted but celebrated. Let's toss aside the shame and guilt that often accompany discussions of solo sexuality. Embrace the idea that your pleasure is a natural, healthy part of who you are. When we share stories and experiences about our own journeys toward self-acceptance, we empower others to do the same. The more we talk about it, the more we normalize it, creating a ripple effect that encourages everyone to explore their own pleasures without fear.

Intimacy, even in solo practices, is deeply personal and varies from person to person. Some may find intimacy through a soft, reflective approach, while others might revel in a more intense, adventurous style. The key is to honor your unique rhythm and preferences. Take the time to connect with your body, listen to its whispers, and respond lovingly. Remember, intimacy is not just about physical sensations; it's about creating a safe space for your desires and fantasies to flourish, making every moment of self-pleasure an act of self-love.

Celebrate the empowerment that comes from reclaiming your body and your pleasure. By embracing the diversity in how we experience pleasure, we not only enrich our own lives but also contribute to a broader cultural shift that values each individual's journey. Self-pleasure is not merely an act; it's a statement of autonomy and joy. So, raise a toast to the wonderful variety of experiences that make up our sexual lives. Each exploration is a step toward mastering pleasure, where everyone's unique expression adds to the beautiful mosaic of human sexuality.

Empowerment Through Knowledge

Knowledge is the ultimate key to unlocking the doors of pleasure, especially when it comes to self-exploration. The journey of mastering self-pleasure begins with understanding your own body and its unique responses. It's like embarking on an exciting treasure hunt where the prize is a deeper connection to yourself. As you dive into the world of solo sexual practices, the more you learn about anatomy, arousal, and your personal preferences, the better equipped you are to create experiences that are not just pleasurable but transformative. So, grab your metaphorical compass and let's navigate this delightful terrain.

Consider this: every time you explore a new technique or read about a different approach to self-pleasure, you're adding a new color to your palette. You aren't just going through the motions; you are crafting a masterpiece of your own intimate experiences. Understanding the various ways your body can respond to different stimuli allows for an explosion of sensations that can make your solo sessions not just enjoyable but exhilarating. Whether it's experimenting with different rhythms, pressures, or even the type of lubricant, knowledge empowers you to customize your pleasure to fit your unique desires.

Breaking societal taboos is another crucial aspect of this journey. For too long, discussions about masturbation and self-pleasure have been shrouded in shame and secrecy. But knowledge is your shield against these outdated notions. By educating yourself and engaging in open conversations about self-pleasure, you reclaim your right to enjoy intimacy with yourself without guilt or hesitation. This empowerment isn't just personal; it creates a ripple effect that encourages others to embrace their desires, fostering a community where pleasure is celebrated rather than stigmatized.

It's not all about techniques and tips, though. Mental health plays a significant role in your ability to enjoy self-pleasure fully. Understanding the connection between a healthy mind and a fulfilled sexual life is essential. Knowledge about how stress, anxiety, or past traumas can affect your relationship with pleasure allows you to cultivate a more supportive inner dialogue. When you empower yourself with this understanding, you open the door to healing and reclaiming your body as a source of joy, rather than a battleground of insecurities.

The journey of empowerment through knowledge is about embracing your individuality and celebrating your desires. Every fact you learn, every technique you master, and every taboo you shatter adds to your self-discovery. So, let that playful spirit guide you as you delve into the world of solo sexual practices. It's about more than just pleasure; it's about crafting a fulfilling relationship with yourself, one that honors your needs and desires. So go forth, explore, and let your curiosity lead the way to a more empowered and pleasurable life.

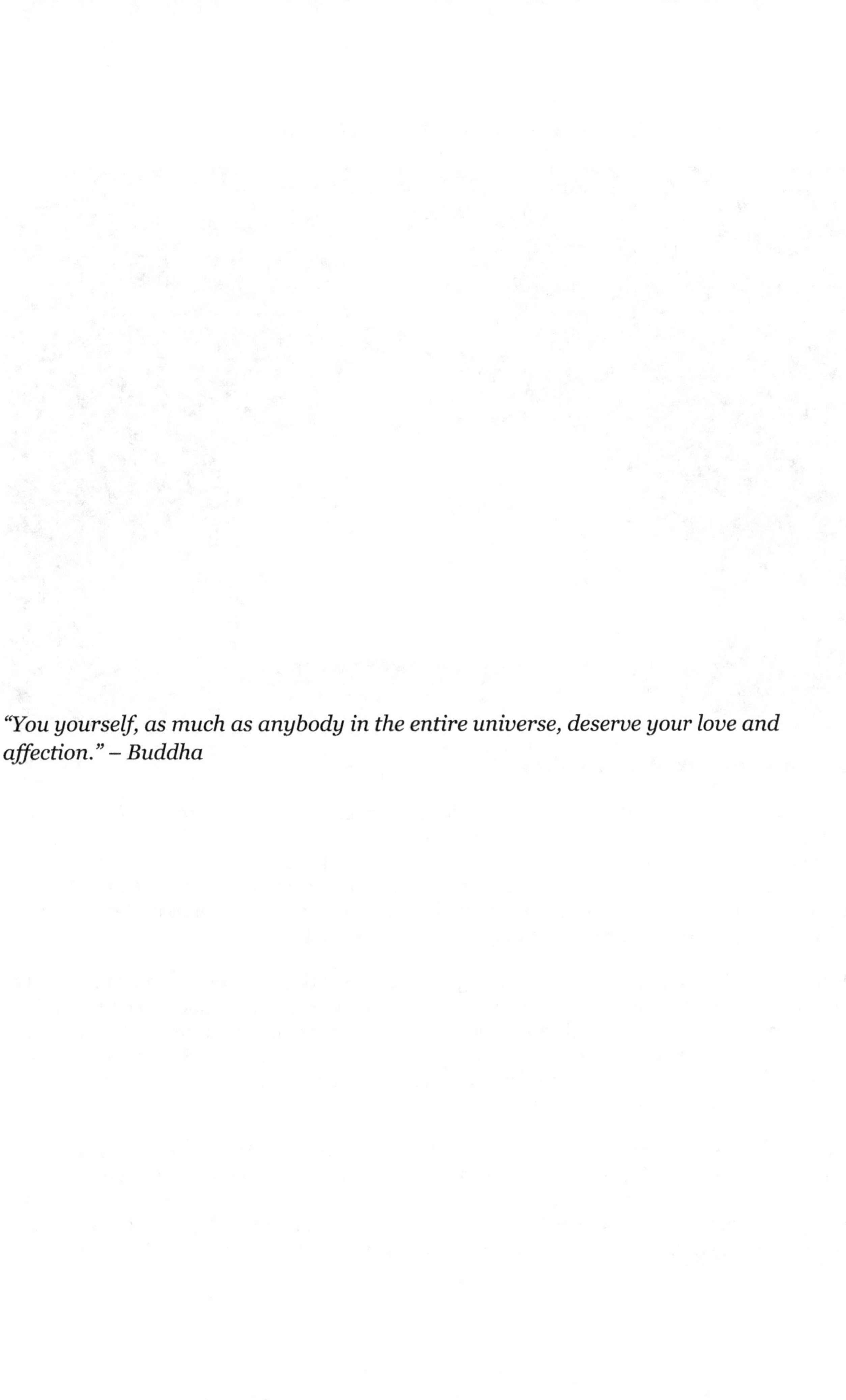

"You yourself, as much as anybody in the entire universe, deserve your love and affection." – Buddha

Chapter 7: Navigating Emotions and Mental Health

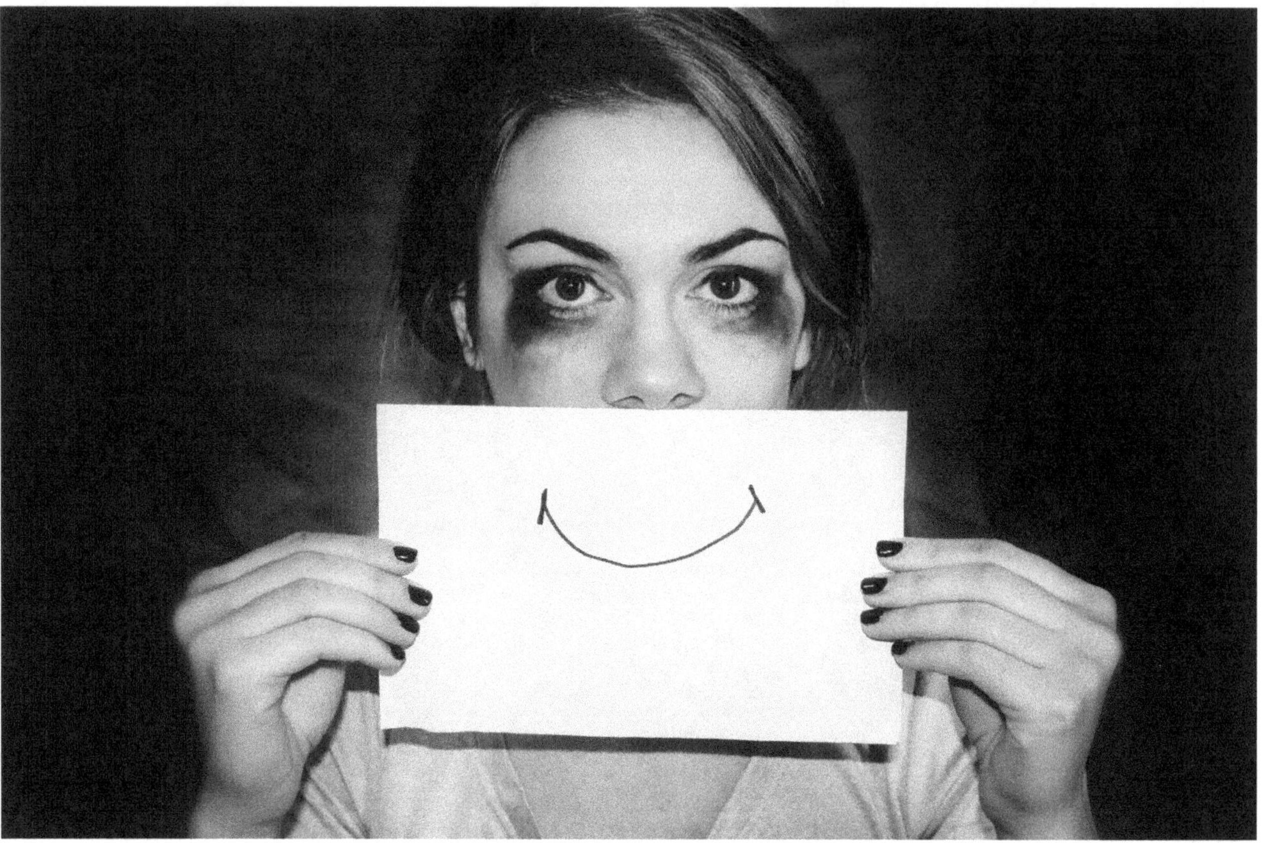

Pleasure as a Tool for Healing

Imagine this: you're feeling stressed, overwhelmed, or simply out of sorts. What if I told you that the key to lifting your spirits and nurturing your mind could be found in the most delightful and personal of experiences? That's right! Pleasure, especially when it comes to solo sexual practices, can be a powerful tool for healing. Engaging in self-pleasure isn't just about physical gratification; it's a joyous journey into understanding your body, your desires, and ultimately, your mental well-being.

When we talk about pleasure as a healing tool, it's essential to recognize how intimately connected our minds and bodies truly are. Masturbation is not a taboo topic reserved for whispers and secrecy; it's a vibrant expression of self-love and acceptance. By exploring your body, you uncover not only the spots that bring you joy but also the emotions tied to those sensations. Letting go and surrendering to the pleasure can offer a cathartic release, helping you process feelings that might otherwise linger like unwanted guests.

Now, let's dive into the science of it all! When you engage in self-pleasure, your body releases a cocktail of feel-good hormones like dopamine and oxytocin. These natural mood lifters can help alleviate anxiety and stress, giving you a much-needed boost. It's like your own personal spa day, but instead of fancy oils and soothing music, you have the vibrant rhythm of your own heartbeat and the electrifying sensations that come with exploring your body. By making time for these solo sessions, you're not just indulging; you're investing in your mental health.

Breaking societal taboos surrounding self-pleasure opens up a world where empowerment reigns. Imagine a community where we celebrate our bodies and embrace our desires without shame. When we learn to reclaim our pleasure, we dismantle the false narratives that have kept us from fully connecting with ourselves. This journey reminds us that pleasure is not something to be earned or negotiated—it is a natural part of being human, a birthright that cultivates intimacy with ourselves.

Mastering pleasure can lead to a deeper understanding and appreciation of our sexual lives. The techniques you explore during these solo sessions not only enhance your personal experience but can also enrich your connections with others. By becoming attuned to your own needs and desires, you're better equipped to communicate them in intimate relationships. So, let's celebrate pleasure as a healing tool, one self-discovery adventure at a time! Embrace the journey, and let your body guide you toward joy and empowerment.

Understanding Your Feelings

Understanding your feelings is like peeling back the layers of a deliciously complex fruit. Each layer reveals something new, something juicy, and sometimes a little tangy. When it comes to self-pleasure and masturbation, our feelings can be a whirlwind of excitement, guilt, curiosity, and empowerment. Embracing this emotional landscape is essential for deepening your connection with yourself and enhancing your solo sexual practices. So, let's dive into those feelings and explore what they mean for you and your pleasure journey.

First, let's talk about the thrill. That rush of excitement when you think about indulging in self-pleasure is a feeling worth celebrating. It's not just about the act; it's about the anticipation, the build-up, and the joyous exploration of your own body. Allow yourself to revel in that feeling! Whether it's a cheeky thought that brings a smirk to your face or the tingle of desire that dances down your spine, acknowledging these sensations can unlock a treasure trove of pleasure. Remember, pleasure is a natural part of being human, and feeling excited about it is a beautiful thing.

But what about the not-so-fun feelings? Guilt and shame often sneak in, courtesy of societal taboos that have been ingrained in us since childhood. It's time to kick those pesky feelings to the curb! Understanding why you feel guilty or ashamed can be liberating. Are these feelings rooted in outdated beliefs or messages you received growing up? By questioning and reframing these thoughts, you can reclaim your body and your pleasure. Embrace the idea that your feelings are valid, and every emotion contributes to your unique experience of self-exploration.

As you navigate your feelings, don't forget the power of self-compassion. It's easy to be hard on yourself—especially when you're exploring something as intimate as masturbation. Instead of judging your feelings, treat them as old friends visiting for tea. Invite them in, listen to their stories, and let them know they're welcome. This playful approach allows you to be gentle with yourself, making space for vulnerability and authenticity. After all, self-pleasure is about celebrating who you are, and that includes every delightful and messy feeling that comes with it.

Embracing your feelings can lead to a deeper understanding of your desires and needs. As you explore your emotional landscape, you'll discover what truly excites you and what holds you back. This self-awareness is crucial for enhancing your solo sexual practices and mastering techniques that resonate with you. By understanding your feelings, you empower yourself to create a fulfilling sexual life that honors your unique journey. So go ahead, dive into those feelings! They're not just there to be understood; they're there to guide you towards the delicious pleasure you deserve.

Self-Care and Aftercare

Self-care and aftercare are essential components of the self-exploration journey, particularly when diving into the world of solo sexual practices and masturbation techniques. Just like any thrilling adventure, the exploration of one's own body and pleasure can leave you feeling exhilarated and, at times, a little spent. Think of self-care as the cozy blanket you wrap around yourself after a wild escapade, providing comfort and rejuvenation. It's all about creating a loving space where you can celebrate your discoveries, reflect on your experiences, and nurture your mental health.

First things first: embrace the post-pleasure glow. After a session of self-exploration, take a moment to savor that delightful feeling. This is your time to bask in the afterglow, where your body is buzzing with pleasure and your mind is alight with new insights. Perhaps you want to journal about what you experienced or what techniques brought you the most joy. Writing can be a playful way to reconnect with your emotions and thoughts, allowing you to process the experience while celebrating your body's capabilities. So grab a colorful pen and let your imagination run wild!

Next, consider a little pampering to elevate your self-care routine. This could be as simple as enjoying a warm bath infused with your favorite essential oils or treating yourself to a soothing cup of herbal tea. You might even want to indulge in some delicious snacks that make you feel good. The goal here is to engage in activities that enhance your well-being and make you feel cherished. Remember, self-care isn't just about physical touch; it encompasses mental and emotional nourishment too! So go ahead, create a mini spa day at home or dance around your living room with your favorite tunes.

Aftercare is particularly important when exploring your sexual self. It can be a time to ground yourself, reconnect with your body, and integrate your experience. Consider cuddling up with a soft blanket and watching a feel-good movie or practicing some gentle stretches that honor your body. This phase is all about listening to what your body needs and responding with kindness. Whether it's a moment of silence to reflect, a chat with a trusted friend, or even some playful self-massage, nurturing yourself after a pleasure session helps reinforce that you are worthy of love and care.

Don't underestimate the power of community and conversation in your self-care journey. Engaging with others who share your interests can help break down societal taboos surrounding self-pleasure and intimacy. Join discussions online or in person where you can share experiences, techniques, and tips. This sense of connection can amplify your empowerment, making you feel supported and understood. Remember, self-care and aftercare aren't just about what you do alone; they can also thrive within a community that celebrates pleasure, intimacy, and the beautiful journey of reclaiming your body and your joy.

"Learning to honor your own pleasure is one of the most radical acts of self-care you can practice." – Adrienne Maree Brown

Chapter 8: Expanding Your Repertoire

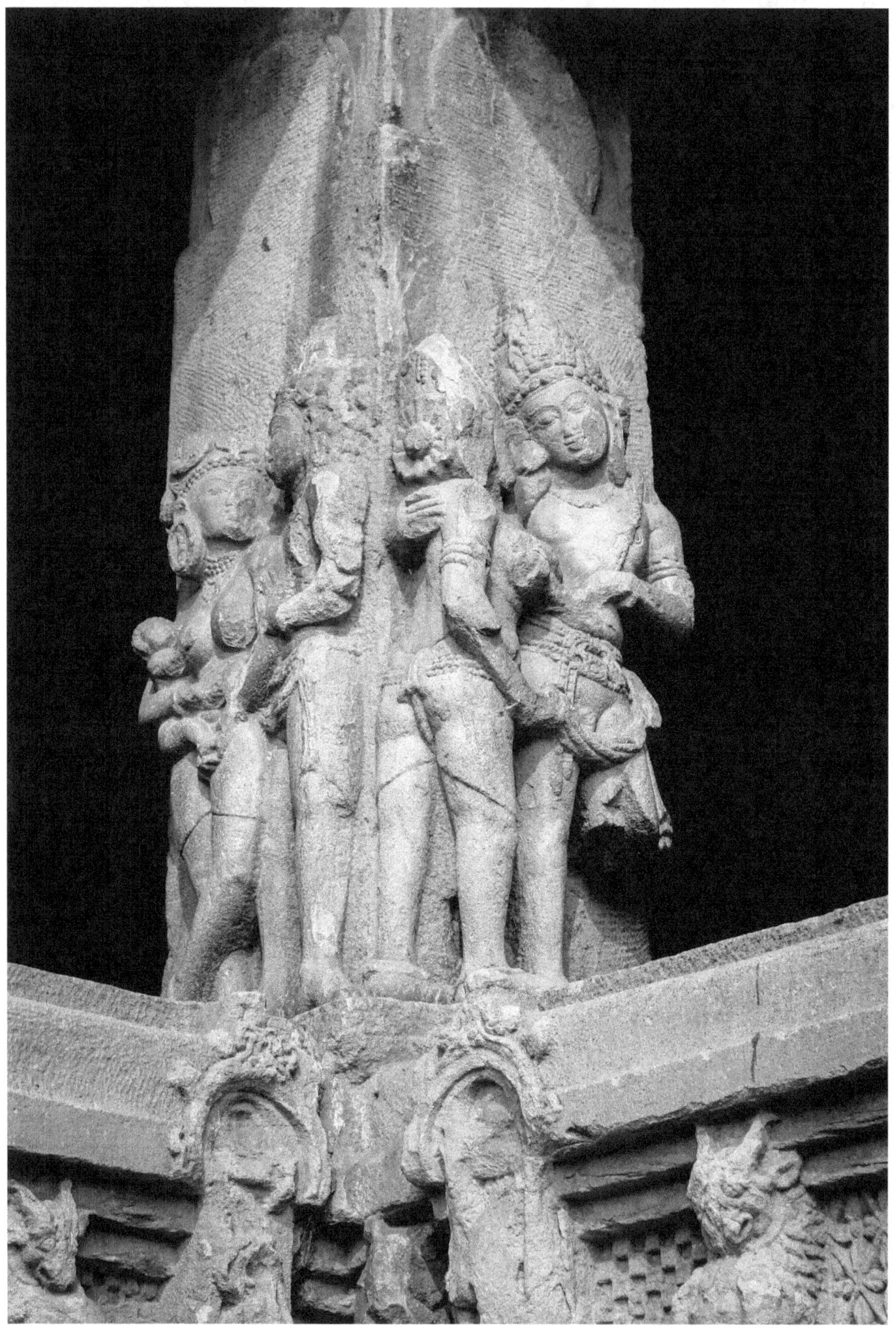

New Techniques to Try

Exploring new techniques in the realm of self-pleasure can be a thrilling adventure that unlocks deeper layers of intimacy with your own body. Embracing the playful side of solo sexual practices can lead to discovering sensations you never knew existed. Imagine embarking on a journey where curiosity guides you, and every touch becomes an invitation to explore. In this delightful dance with yourself, creativity is your best friend, and the only limits are those of your imagination.

One exciting technique to try is the "Sensory Exploration" method. Gather a variety of objects with different textures—from soft feathers to silky fabrics, or even playful sponges. As you indulge in the sensations these items provide, allow yourself to get lost in the experience. Focus fully on how each texture feels against your skin, paying attention to your body's responses. This not only heightens your awareness but also creates a rich tapestry of feelings that can elevate your pleasure to new heights.

Consider incorporating elements of mindfulness into your solo sessions through the "Breath and Flow" technique. Start by finding a comfortable position and take a few deep, grounding breaths. Allow each inhale to fill you with warmth and openness, while each exhale releases any tension you may be holding. As you begin to explore your body, synchronize your movements with your breath. This connection not only enhances physical pleasure but also fosters a deeper emotional connection with yourself, making the experience more fulfilling.

Another playful approach is the "Fantasy Journaling" technique. Before diving into your practice, spend some time writing down your fantasies or desires in a journal. Let your imagination run wild and don't hold back! Once you've penned your thoughts, use them as a guide during your self-pleasure session. This creative expression can ignite your arousal and transport you into a world where anything is possible. As you bring your fantasies to life, you'll not only enjoy the physical sensations but also cultivate a profound sense of empowerment and self-acceptance.

Finally, don't shy away from the world of technology. Explore the realm of sex toys and apps designed to enhance solo pleasure. Whether it's a sleek vibrator or an interactive app that offers guided sessions, these tools can add an exciting twist to your routine. Experiment with different devices to find what resonates with you, and don't forget to mix and match techniques. The key is to keep your exploration lively and fun, so embrace your playful spirit and allow your body to lead the way. Each new technique you try is a step toward mastering your pleasure, breaking free from societal taboos, and ultimately reclaiming your body in the most joyous way possible.

Incorporating Toys and Accessories

Incorporating toys and accessories into your solo sexual practices can transform the experience from ordinary to extraordinary. Imagine the thrill of adding a little buzz or a tantalizing texture to your self-exploration sessions. Whether it's a sleek vibrator, a soft feather, or even some playful blindfolds, these items can help you discover new sensations and elevate your pleasure. The right accessory can turn a routine act into a delightful journey, allowing you to tap into your desires and push the boundaries of your pleasure.

When it comes to choosing toys, the world is your oyster! From classic vibrators to innovative clitoral stimulators, there's an endless variety to explore. Consider what excites you the most. Are you drawn to something with a bit of power? Or maybe you prefer a gentle touch that caresses rather than overwhelms. Don't shy away from experimenting with different materials and shapes. Silicone, glass, or even metal can offer unique sensations that can deepen your connection with your body. The key is to let curiosity guide you and to embrace the playful spirit of exploration.

Accessories can also enhance your solo sessions in ways you might not have considered. Think about incorporating elements like scented candles, soft music, or even a cozy blanket to create an inviting atmosphere. These additions can heighten your senses and help you relax into the experience. Lighting can also play a significant role—soft, dim lighting can evoke a sense of intimacy that allows you to feel more connected to yourself. Remember, self-pleasure is not just a physical act; it's an opportunity to indulge in a holistic experience that nourishes both body and mind.

Don't forget about the power of fantasy in your solo play! Toys can be the perfect companions in bringing your wildest dreams to life. Consider role-playing scenarios or exploring themes that excite you. You might find that a particular toy can help you embody different characters or vibes, turning your self-exploration into an empowering performance. This playful approach can help break societal taboos around self-pleasure, allowing you to reclaim your narrative and celebrate your desires without judgment.

Always remember that the journey of self-discovery through toys and accessories is uniquely yours. There are no right or wrong ways to explore, and what works for one person might not resonate with another. The most important aspect is to enjoy the process and to listen to your body. Celebrate each step, whether it's a new technique, a toy that makes you giggle, or a moment of pure bliss. Embrace the joy of playfulness, and allow yourself to fully experience the empowerment that comes from mastering your own pleasure.

Solo Play and Creativity

Solo play is often viewed through a narrow lens, typically shrouded in secrecy or a sense of shame. However, it can be one of the most liberating forms of self-expression, allowing individuals to explore their bodies and desires without the constraints of societal expectations. Engaging in solo play opens a door to a world of creativity, where the only limits are those set by your own imagination. It's a canvas where you can paint your fantasies, experiment with sensations, and discover what truly brings you pleasure, all while enjoying the unique opportunity to connect deeply with yourself.

When you embark on the journey of solo play, think of it as a creative playground. You can mix and match techniques, tools, and settings to find what tickles your fancy. Whether it's using different types of lubrication, experimenting with temperature play, or incorporating toys, the possibilities are endless. This is your chance to break free from the conventional, to step into a realm where you are the sole architect of your pleasure. With each session, you become more attuned to your body, learning what makes you tick and what sparks joy in your intimate encounters.

Exploring solo play also aids in enhancing your mental health. In a world that often bombards us with unrealistic body images and societal norms, taking time to prioritize your pleasure can be an act of radical self-love. It allows you to reclaim your body, celebrating its uniqueness and capabilities. As you indulge in self-pleasure, you send powerful messages to your brain that reinforce positive body image and self-acceptance. This, in turn, can lead to reduced anxiety and increased confidence, both in and out of the bedroom.

Moreover, solo play fosters a profound sense of intimacy with yourself. It's not just about the physical act; it's a journey into your psyche, uncovering desires and fantasies that may have been tucked away for too long. This intimate relationship with yourself lays the foundation for healthier connections with others. When you understand your own needs and desires, you can communicate them more effectively in partnered experiences. Solo play becomes a nurturing space where you can cultivate a rich understanding of what intimacy means to you.

Embracing solo play as a creative outlet allows you to challenge societal taboos surrounding masturbation and self-exploration. By openly discussing and celebrating these practices, you contribute to a culture that champions sexual wellness and empowerment. You become an advocate for breaking down the barriers that have long suppressed the joy of self-pleasure. So, let your creativity run wild; explore, experiment, and indulge in the delightful journey of solo play. After all, mastering your pleasure is not just about the act itself, but about the joy of discovering who you truly are.

"When you connect with yourself, you unlock the power to transform every relationship in your life, starting with the one you have within." – Yung Pueblo

Chapter 9: Reclaiming Your Pleasure

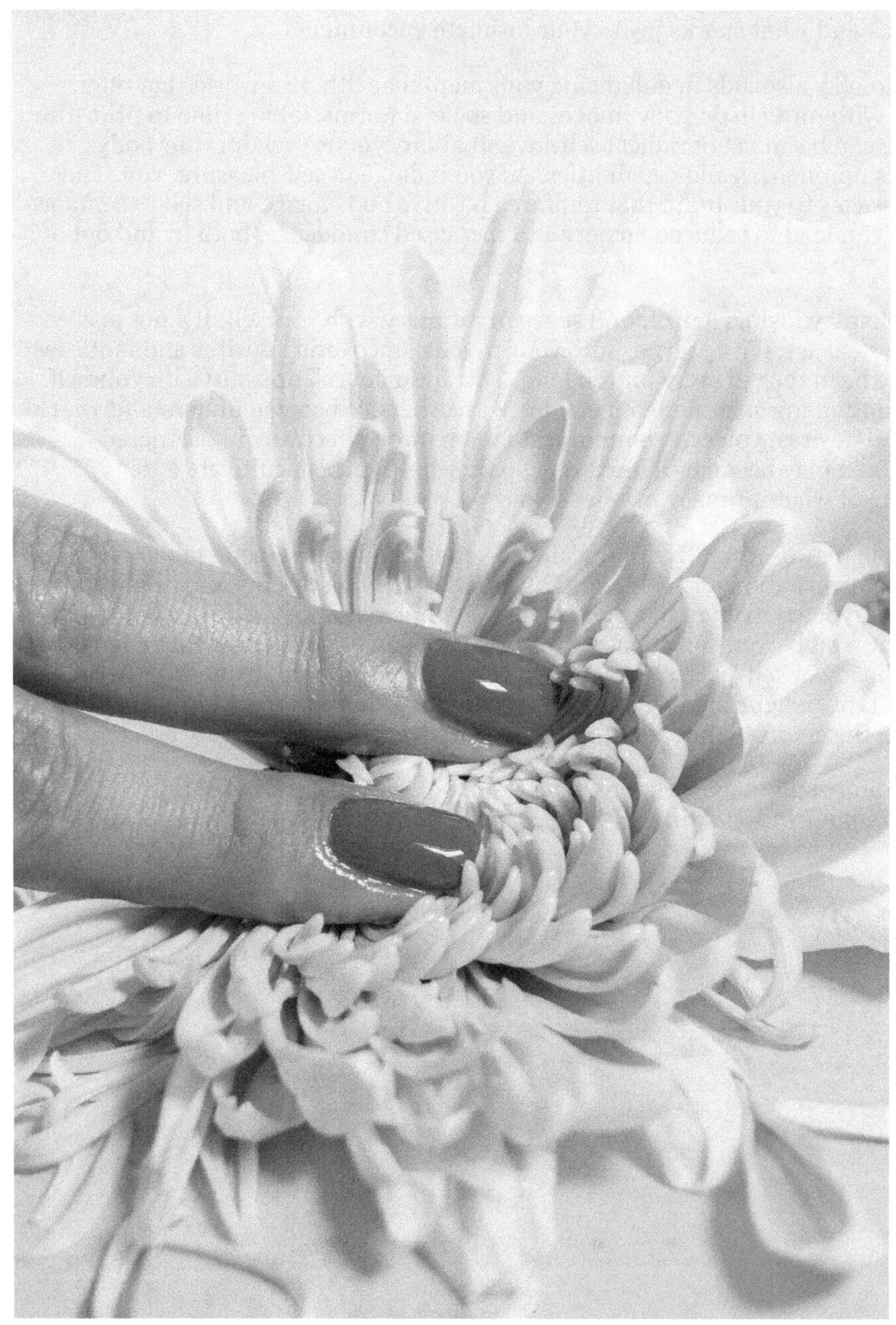

Fostering a Positive Mindset

Fostering a positive mindset is the secret ingredient to unlocking the full potential of your solo sexual practices. Just like a delicious recipe, the right attitude can transform the ordinary into the extraordinary. When you approach self-pleasure with an open heart and a curious spirit, you invite joy and exploration into your intimate moments. It's about embracing your desires without judgment and allowing yourself the freedom to discover what brings you pleasure. So, let go of any lingering guilt or shame; it's time to celebrate your body and all the delightful sensations it can offer.

To cultivate this positive mindset, start by engaging in self-affirmation. Look in the mirror and remind yourself of your worthiness and desirability. Compliment your body, not just for how it looks, but for everything it does. Remember, your body is not merely a vessel; it's a playground of pleasure waiting to be explored. By recognizing your unique beauty and embracing your individuality, you create a solid foundation for a pleasurable experience. Self-love is the ultimate power move, and it sets the stage for an empowered journey of self-discovery.

Next, let's sprinkle in some playful curiosity. Approach your solo sessions with the same enthusiasm you'd bring to a new adventure. Experiment with different techniques, explore various sensations, and don't shy away from trying something new. Whether it's incorporating toys, changing up your routine, or even exploring new fantasies, the world of self-pleasure is vast and exciting. Every experience is a chance to learn more about your desires and boundaries. Remember, there are no right or wrong ways to enjoy your body—only opportunities to discover what feels best for you.

Additionally, it's essential to create a sacred space for your intimate explorations. Design a cozy nook that feels inviting and safe, where you can unwind and focus solely on your pleasure. Surround yourself with items that inspire relaxation, like soft lighting, soothing music, or even aromatic candles. This space can become your personal sanctuary, encouraging a positive mindset that enhances your experiences. When you treat your self-pleasure time as a cherished ritual, it transforms into something truly special, elevating your mood and reinforcing the connection between your mind and body.

Now, let go of societal expectations and embrace your own narrative around pleasure. The journey to mastering self-pleasure is uniquely yours, and it's time to reclaim your story. A positive mindset means recognizing that pleasure is not just a taboo topic; it's a natural part of life. By embracing your desires and sharing your experiences—whether through conversations with friends or in supportive communities—you contribute to breaking down the barriers that society has built around intimacy. Celebrate your journey, uplift others, and together, let's foster a culture where pleasure and self-love are celebrated as the beautiful, empowering experiences they truly are.

Celebrating Your Journey

Celebrating your journey in self-pleasure is like throwing a confetti party for your own personal growth. Each step you take towards understanding your body and desires deserves a moment of recognition. When you embrace the path of self-exploration, you're not just indulging in pleasure; you're also engaging in a life-affirming practice that fosters empowerment and self-love. So, let's break out the balloons and streamers because your journey is worth celebrating!

As you navigate the world of solo sexual practices, it's essential to acknowledge the milestones along the way. Perhaps you've discovered a new technique that sends shivers down your spine, or maybe you've learned to appreciate your body in ways you never thought possible. Each of these moments is a victory, a stepping stone towards deeper intimacy with yourself. Take a moment to reflect on these triumphs, however small they may seem. They contribute to the bigger picture of your sexual liberation and self-acceptance.

Engaging in self-pleasure isn't just about the physical act; it's a celebration of your intimate relationship with yourself. It's a canvas for creativity, allowing you to explore what brings you joy and satisfaction. Whether it's experimenting with different techniques or discovering new erogenous zones, each experience adds to the vibrant tapestry of your sexual life. So, don't shy away from adding a splash of color to your practice! Dance, laugh, and let yourself be whimsical in the process.

To truly celebrate your journey, it's important to break away from societal taboos that may have held you back. Many of us grow up with messages that shame our natural desires, but now is the time to flip the script. Reclaim your body and your pleasure with exuberance! Surround yourself with affirmations that honor your journey and remind you that your pleasure is not just valid but essential. Shatter those stigmas and replace them with a confetti of self-love and acceptance.

Always remember that this celebration isn't a one-time event; it's an ongoing festival of self-discovery. As you continue to explore and master your solo sexual practices, keep that playful spirit alive. Share your experiences with trusted friends, join communities that uplift and empower, and keep learning about your body and pleasure. Every laugh, every sigh, and every moment of bliss is part of a grand celebration that honors who you are and who you're becoming. So go ahead, raise a glass to yourself and get ready for the next chapter in your delightful journey of self-pleasure!

Encouraging Self-Expression

Encouraging self-expression is like opening the door to a vibrant world where your desires and fantasies can dance freely. This journey is all about embracing who you are, both physically and emotionally. Think of self-expression as your personal playground, where each swing, slide, and merry-go-round represents a different facet of your pleasure. By tapping into your unique self, you can unlock the full potential of your solo sexual practices, transforming what might feel like a guilty secret into an exhilarating celebration of your body and mind.

When it comes to self-pleasure, the first step is to break free from the shackles of societal expectations. Many of us have been conditioned to believe that talking about our desires is taboo or that pleasure is something to be hushed away. But let's flip the script!

Self-expression is your rebellion against these outdated norms. It's time to take ownership of your pleasure and express it in ways that feel right for you. Whether it's through writing, art, or simply vocalizing your desires, letting your thoughts flow can be liberating and empowering.

Visualize your ideal self-care routine, and don't shy away from incorporating playful elements. Think of scented candles, soft music, or even a cozy blanket that makes you feel safe and cherished. These little touches set the stage for exploration. As you dive deeper into your solo sexual practices, remember to listen to your body. Each sigh, shiver, and flutter is a form of self-expression. Allow yourself to be curious about what feels good, and don't be afraid to experiment with different techniques, toys, or even fantasy scenarios. This is your time to play, discover, and delight in what makes you tick.

As you continue this journey, consider journaling your experiences. Writing can be a powerful tool for self-reflection and growth. Document your feelings, your triumphs, and the moments of pure joy you discover through self-exploration. Not only does this practice enhance your self-awareness, but it also creates a space for you to articulate your desires and boundaries. By putting pen to paper, you're giving voice to your inner world, making it easier to explore what you truly want, both in and out of the bedroom.

Each step you take towards embracing your pleasure is a victory worth shouting from the rooftops. Share your newfound confidence and insights with supportive friends or communities that celebrate empowerment and body positivity. Encourage others to join in this playful exploration of self-discovery. Together, you can create a ripple effect that breaks down barriers and inspires everyone to reclaim their bodies and their pleasure. Remember, the more you express yourself, the more vibrant and fulfilling your sexual life becomes. So go ahead—play, discover, and revel in the joy of self-expression!

"Your body is your sacred space. Treat it with reverence, listen to its needs, and give it the love it deserves." – Monica Lynne Chase

Chapter 10: Beyond the Solo Experience

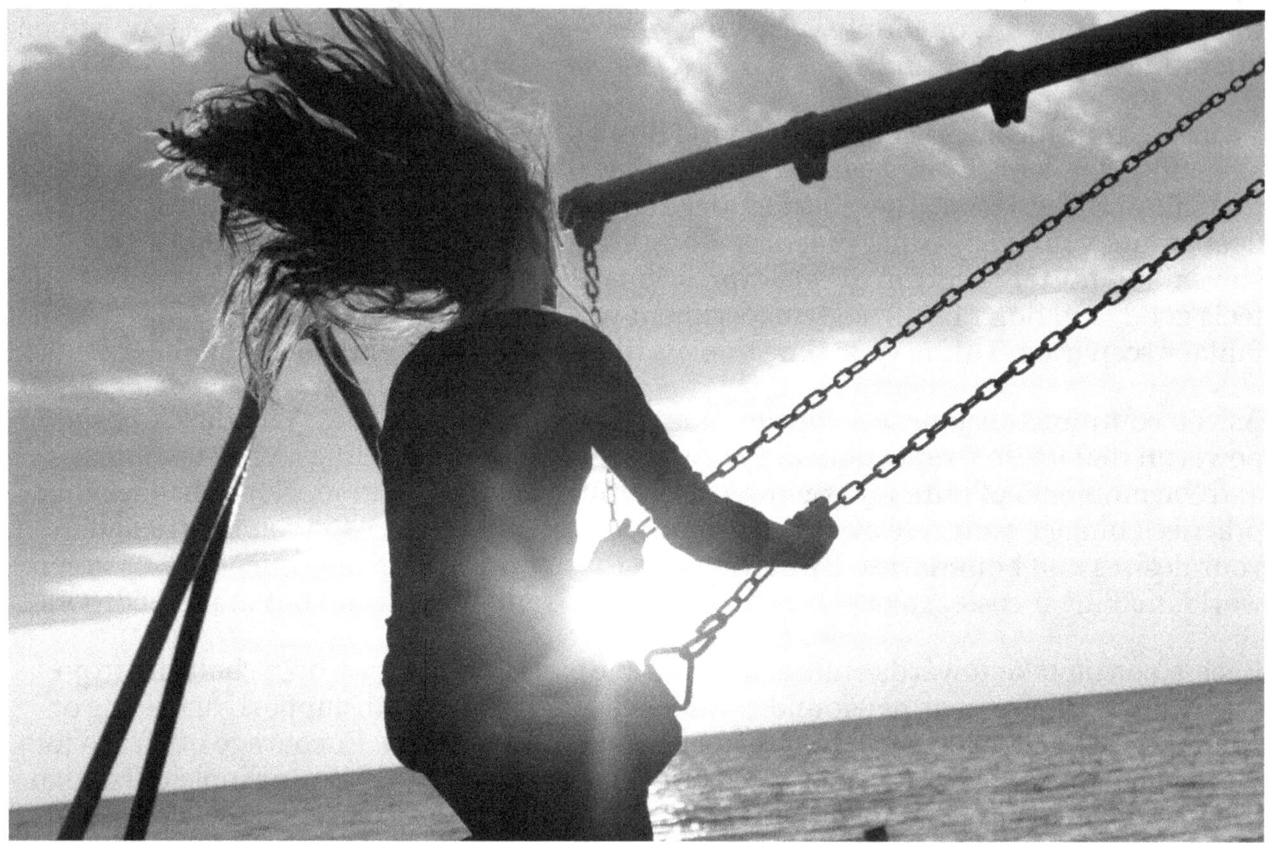

Integrating Pleasure into Daily Life

Integrating pleasure into daily life is like sprinkling a little fairy dust on the mundane. Imagine transforming your routine into a delightful dance of self-discovery, where each moment is an invitation to explore the realms of your body and desires. It's all about shifting your perspective and allowing pleasure to seep into the crevices of your day, turning the ordinary into the extraordinary. Whether it's setting aside a few moments to connect with your breath or indulging in a luxurious bubble bath, these small pleasures can become powerful rituals that celebrate your body and your desires.

Start your day with intention. As you wake up, take a moment to appreciate your body—feel the sheets against your skin, stretch out, and breathe deeply. This simple act of mindfulness can create a foundation for pleasure throughout your day. Why not add a playful twist to your morning routine? Consider incorporating a few sensual movements or a quick dance to your favorite song. This isn't just about getting your heart racing; it's about awakening your senses and inviting joy into your life from the very start.

Midday is a perfect time for a pleasure break. Instead of scrolling through your phone or grabbing a quick snack, take a few moments to engage with your body. Try a quick solo pleasure practice, even if it's just for a few minutes. Explore what feels good—whether it's gentle touches or imagining sensual scenarios. This isn't just about physical pleasure; it's a way to reconnect with yourself, release tension, and remind yourself that pleasure is your birthright. Breaking the societal taboo around self-exploration can transform these moments into empowering acts of self-love.

As the sun sets, create a sensual atmosphere in your space. Dim the lights, light a candle, or play soft music that stirs your soul. This is your time to unwind and indulge in whatever brings you joy. Whether it's a warm bath, a favorite book, or indulging in a little self-stimulation, make it a point to savor this time. Embrace the power of your fantasies, allowing them to ignite your imagination and enhance your intimacy with yourself. It's not just about physical pleasure; it's about nurturing your mental well-being and embracing your desires without shame.

Integrate pleasure into your social interactions. Share your journey with friends or engage in conversations that challenge societal norms around pleasure and intimacy. Consider hosting a gathering where everyone can explore their own forms of self-pleasure in a safe space. This can be a liberating experience, allowing you and your friends to break taboos and celebrate your bodies together. When you invite pleasure into every facet of your life, you empower yourself and those around you to reclaim their joy, intimacy, and connection to self. Remember, pleasure isn't just a destination; it's a joyful journey that begins with you.

Sharing Your Journey with Others

Sharing your journey with others can be as liberating as the journey itself. When we open up about our experiences with self-pleasure and intimacy, we not only empower ourselves but also create a ripple effect that encourages others to explore their own paths. Imagine the joy of discussing your favorite solo sexual practices with a friend, swapping tips on techniques and discovering new ways to reclaim pleasure. Just like a secret club, sharing these experiences can foster a sense of community and help break down those pesky societal taboos that often keep us silent.

Think about the last time you had a candid conversation about your sexual life. Wasn't it refreshing to dive deep into the intricacies of what brings you joy? By sharing your journey, you invite others to reflect on their experiences, creating a safe space where vulnerability thrives. Whether it's over coffee or a cozy chat online, discussing self-pleasure opens the door to understanding that intimacy is not just about partners; it's about nurturing a relationship with yourself. Embrace the playful side of these discussions, and you'll find that laughter and curiosity are the best companions on this exploration.

One of the most delightful aspects of sharing your journey is the potential for learning and growth. You may have stumbled upon a technique that transformed your experience, and by sharing it, you could spark a lightbulb moment for someone else. Imagine your friend trying out your favorite solo sexual practice and discovering a new level of pleasure they never knew existed. This exchange of knowledge not only enhances personal experiences but also strengthens connections, as you support each other in embracing your sexuality.

As you share, remember that it's not just about the techniques or the physical aspects of pleasure. It's also about the mental health benefits that come from being open and honest about your desires. By discussing your journey, you can highlight how self-pleasure contributes to emotional well-being, boosting confidence and promoting a healthier relationship with your body. When we normalize these conversations, we dismantle the stigma that has long surrounded topics of self-care and intimacy, making room for empowerment and self-acceptance.

In this playful exploration of sharing your journey, don't forget to celebrate the milestones, big and small. Whether it's finding a new favorite technique or simply feeling more comfortable in your skin, every step counts. By sharing these victories, you inspire others to take their own leaps of faith. Let your story be a beacon of hope and encouragement, reminding everyone that embracing pleasure is not only a personal journey but a shared adventure that we can all enjoy together.

Continuing the Exploration

Continuing the exploration of self-pleasure is like stepping into a magical realm where your body is the ultimate playground. Imagine yourself as an intrepid explorer, armed with curiosity and a sense of adventure, ready to uncover the hidden treasures of your own desires. Every time you engage in solo sexual practices, you're not just indulging in a moment of pleasure; you're embarking on a journey of self-discovery. Whether it's through a gentle caress or an exhilarating technique, each experience allows you to peel back layers of societal conditioning, reclaiming your right to pleasure.

As you delve deeper into the art of masturbation, think of it as a delightful dance with your own body. Each move, each touch, is an invitation to explore the rhythm that feels right for you. You might find yourself experimenting with different techniques, from the classic to the adventurous, discovering what truly brings you joy. Remember, there are no wrong ways to enjoy yourself—every exploration is valid and worthy of celebration. Embrace the playful spirit of experimentation, and let your body guide you through this exhilarating journey.

Don't shy away from incorporating tools and toys into your solo sessions. They can add a whole new dimension to your exploration. Whether it's a soft feather for teasing or a more sophisticated gadget that promises waves of pleasure, these tools can enhance your experience and help you uncover new heights of satisfaction. Just as every explorer needs the right equipment, you too can arm yourself with a toolkit of pleasure that makes your adventures even more enjoyable. Be bold, be daring, and let your imagination run wild.

Mental health plays a crucial role in the journey of self-exploration. As you engage in solo sexual practices, you may find that they not only bring physical pleasure but also act as a powerful form of self-care. Taking the time to connect with your body can help release pent-up emotions, reduce stress, and boost your overall well-being. Embrace these moments as sacred time for yourself, where you can unwind and nourish your spirit. This connection between pleasure and mental health is a beautiful reminder that caring for yourself is a fundamental part of living a fulfilling life.

Continuing the exploration of your body and pleasure is a liberating act that defies societal taboos. By owning your pleasure, you are not just reclaiming your body; you are making a bold statement about your right to experience joy. So go ahead, dance to your own rhythm, explore every inch of your landscape, and indulge in the pleasure that is inherently yours. Each session is a chance to affirm your identity, celebrate your desires, and empower yourself. Let the exploration continue, and may each moment be filled with joy, discovery, and unabashed pleasure.

"True freedom lies in embracing all parts of yourself, unapologetically and with compassion." – Brene Brown

Resources

Here's a comprehensive list of resources for further exploration on self-pleasure, self-love, and sexual wellness. This includes recommended reading, apps, online catalogs, and medical journals that can deepen understanding and support continued growth.

Further Reading

1. Come As You Are: The Surprising New Science That Will Transform Your Sex Life by Emily Nagoski
This book delves into the science of sexuality and pleasure, offering insights on how to embrace your body, desires, and unique pleasure experiences.
2. The Body Keeps the Score: Brain, Mind, and Body in the Healing of Trauma by Bessel van der Kolk
Although focused on trauma, this book addresses how body awareness, including pleasure, can be a tool for healing and self-empowerment.
3. Sex for One: The Joy of Self-Loving by Betty Dodson
Dodson's classic text explores the power of self-pleasure, breaking down barriers and stigmas, and encouraging a joyful, shame-free experience.
4. Better Sex Through Mindfulness by Lori Brotto
This book explores the connection between mindfulness and sexuality, offering research-backed methods to deepen pleasure and presence.
5. Urban Tantra: Sacred Sex for the Twenty-First Century by Barbara Carrellas
Carrellas provides a guide to Tantric practices, blending mindfulness and pleasure, and offering a perspective on the spiritual aspects of self-exploration.

Helpful Apps

1. Ferly
Ferly is a guided app for sexual self-discovery that offers exercises, audio guides, and tools to deepen one's connection with their body and sexuality through mindfulness and empowerment.
2. Mojo
This app focuses on building confidence, offering guided content on solo pleasure, communication, and intimacy.
3. Mjoy
Aimed at encouraging self-love and self-discovery, Mjoy provides a variety of exercises and audio sessions on topics ranging from body acceptance to exploring solo pleasure.
4. Headspace (Mindfulness & Relaxation)

While not specifically focused on sexuality, Headspace offers valuable mindfulness practices that can enhance connection, relaxation, and body awareness.

Online Catalogs and Retailers

1.   Unbound
An inclusive online shop offering products for sexual wellness, self-pleasure, and self-care. Their blog also features articles on solo exploration and sexuality.
2.   Good Vibrations
Known for its welcoming and inclusive approach, Good Vibrations offers a range of educational resources, books, and tools focused on pleasure and empowerment.
3.   Lovehoney
Lovehoney is an international retailer with a vast selection of products and resources on self-exploration, with detailed guides and reviews.
4.   Babeland
An established shop that promotes safe, comfortable, and inclusive products for sexual wellness, Babeland also provides educational materials on topics like body acceptance and solo pleasure.

Medical Journals and Research Articles

1.   The Journal of Sex Research
Published studies on sexuality, including solo pleasure, intimacy, and mental health, providing evidence-based research that explores the impact of self-pleasure on well-being.
2.   Archives of Sexual Behavior
This journal includes research on various aspects of sexual health, including articles on solo pleasure, body positivity, and psychological benefits.
3.   Journal of Sexual Medicine
With peer-reviewed articles, this journal covers a wide range of topics on sexual health, including studies on the physiological and psychological aspects of solo sexuality.
4.   International Journal of Sexual Health
This journal focuses on sexual health and wellness, often addressing solo pleasure as part of a holistic approach to mental and emotional health.
5.   Journal of Sex & Marital Therapy
Offers research articles on self-pleasure, intimacy, and related therapeutic practices, ideal for readers interested in clinical perspectives on sexuality.

A Heartfelt Thank You to My Readers

As you reach the final pages of Mastering Pleasure, I want to extend my deepest gratitude to you for taking this journey with me. This book isn't just a collection of chapters on self-discovery; it's a shared experience, a path paved with curiosity, courage, and the desire for self-love and acceptance. By opening yourself to these pages, you've embraced the power of self-connection, honoring your body and spirit in ways that may once have felt out of reach. Thank you for giving yourself permission to explore, to question, and to celebrate your unique experience of pleasure.

Writing this book has been a journey for me as well—a journey of vulnerability and commitment to creating a space where we can all feel seen, respected, and supported. Knowing that you're here, that you've connected with these words, means everything to me. My hope is that you walk away with not only a deeper understanding of yourself but also a lasting sense of empowerment, acceptance, and love for the person you are.

Remember, this journey doesn't end here. The exploration of self is a lifelong process, one that is as beautiful and complex as you are. Hold close to the knowledge and confidence you've gained, continue to nurture yourself, and never underestimate the importance of your own pleasure and joy. You deserve all of it.

Thank you for allowing me to be part of your journey. May you carry forward a spirit of self-love, curiosity, and endless appreciation for the unique and wonderful person that you are.

Monica Lynne Chase

Fin